The
Monster at
Our Door

The Monster at Our Door

The Global Threat of Avian Flu

Mike Davis

THE NEW PRESS

NEW YORK
LONDON

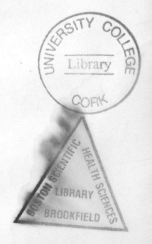

Requests for permission to reproduce selections from this book should be mailed to:
Permissions Department, The New Press, 38 Greene Street, New York, NY 10013.

Published in the United Kingdom by The New Press, New York, 2007
Distributed by Thomson Publishing Services, Ltd

ISBN-13: 978-1-59558-170-9 (pbk)
ISBN-10: 1-59558-170-7 (pbk)
CIP data available

The New Press was established in 1990 as a not-for-profit alternative to the large,
commercial publishing houses currently dominating the book publishing industry. The
New Press operates in the public interest rather than for private gain, and is committed
to publishing, in innovative ways, works of educational, cultural, and community value
that are often deemed insufficiently profitable.

www.thenewpress.com

Printed in the United Kingdom

1   3   5   7   9   10   8   6   4   2

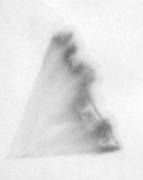

for my comrade doctors:

Michael Alcalay, Stefano Sensi

& Jorge Mancillas

Lo, when the wall is fallen shall it not be said unto you,
Where is the daubing wherewith ye have daubed it?

Ezekiel (xiii, 3, 10–12)

Contents

Contents

The Monster at
Our Door

Preface: Pieta

The evil that happened here in the last month was a sign.[1]

The village chief of Ban Srisomboon

In a time of plague, like the influenza pandemic that swept away my mother's little brother and 40 to 100 million other people in 1918, it is difficult to retain a clear image of individual suffering. Great epidemics, like world wars and famines, massify death into species-level events beyond our emotional comprehension. The afflicted, as a result, die twice: their physical agonies are redoubled by the submergence of their personalities in the black water of megatragedy. As Camus put it, "a dead man has no substance unless one has actually seen him dead; a hundred million corpses broadcast through history are no more than a puff of smoke in the imagination."[2] No one mourns a multitude or keens at the graveside of an abstraction. Unlike certain other social animals, we have no collective sorrow instinct or biological solidarity that is automatically aroused by the destruction of our fellow kind. Indeed, at our worst we find a perverse, often delectable sublimity in Black Deaths, tsunamis, massacres, genocides, and collapsing skyscrapers. In order to grieve over a cataclysm, we must first personify it. The Final Solution, for example, has little gut impact until one reads *The Diary of Anne Frank* or sees the pitiful artifacts in the Holocaust Museum. Then it is possible to weep.

The threat of avian influenza—a plague-in-the-making that the World Health Organization (WHO) fears could kill as many as 100 million people in the next few years—is perhaps most movingly exemplified by the story of Pranee Thongchan and her daughter Sakuntala. Indeed, the image of the dying eleven-year-old tenderly cradled in the arms of her young mother was the *pieta* that gave visceral meaning to the writing of this little book, which reports on the failure of our government and others to protect the world from the imminent danger of an almost unfathomably dangerous influenza outbreak. The intimate and heart-moving scale of this mother-daughter tragedy is precisely what will be lost if avian flu, as so many predict, becomes the next great pestilence of globalization, following in the wake of HIV/AIDS.

Ban Srisomboon is a village of 400 households in Thailand's northern province of Kamphaeng Phet, a pleasant, sleepy region whose decayed temples and palaces attract few tourists but which is renown throughout the country for its famous bananas. Like rural Thais elsewhere, the people of Ban Srisomboon are preoccupied with chickens. They raise free-range poultry for cash income, then invest their earnings in the fighting cocks that are a national obsession. In late August 2004, however, chickens started dying mysteriously throughout the village, much like the rats in Oran in the early scenes of *The Plague*. Unlike the hapless *colons* in Camus's famous novel, however, the farmers of Ban Srisomboon recognized that the dead chickens were a portent of the avian influenza that had been insidiously creeping across Thailand since November 2003.

Given the genetic license-plate number "H5N1" by virologists, this flu subtype had been first recognized in Hong Kong in 1997 when it jumped from waterfowl to humans, killing six of its eighteen victims. A desperate cull of all the poultry in the city contained the first outbreak, but the virus simply went underground, most likely in the "silent reservoir" of domestic ducks. In 2003, it suddenly reappeared on an epic scale throughout China and Southeast Asia. Researchers were horrified to discover that H5N1—like the doomsday bug in Michael Crichton's old thriller, *The Andromeda Strain*—was becoming "progressively more pathogenic" both to chickens and humans. In the first three months of 2004, as new human fatalities were reported from Vietnam and Thailand, more than 120 million chickens and ducks were destroyed in a massive international effort to create a firebreak around the outbreak. Most of the slaughtered poultry belonged to small farmers or contract growers who were often wiped out by the losses. The countryside of Southeast Asia, as a result, was full of apprehension and bitterness.

The family heads of Ban Srisomboon thus faced an excruciating dilemma. On one hand, they were aware that the disease was truly dangerous to their children as well as their chickens and that they were legally required to summon the authorities. On the other hand, they also knew that the government would promptly kill all their poultry, including their prized fighting cocks. The official compensation was only 20 *baht* per bird (about 50 cents), but the cocks were worth up to 10,000 *baht*— in some cases, they were a family's principal wealth.[3]

Bangkok newspapers reported different versions of how the village resolved this contradiction. In one account, the villagers decided to hide the outbreak and hope for the best. In another version, they twice warned the Agriculture Ministry that abnormal numbers of chickens were dying, but officials failed to inspect the village. In any event Sakuntala's uncle, Somsak Laemphakwan, later told reporters that he dug deep holes to ensure that his dead birds did not spread their infection. Despite this precaution, his niece, who like other village children had daily contact with the birds, soon developed a suspicious stomachache and fever. Somsak took her to a nearby clinic, but the nurse dismissed her illness as a bad cold. Five days later, however, Sakuntala began to vomit blood, and she was rushed to the district hospital in the town of Kamphaeng Phet (population 25,000). When she continued to deteriorate, her aunt, Pranom Thongchan, called Sakuntala's mother, who was working in a garment factory near Bangkok, and told her to come home quickly.[4]

Pranee was horrified to discover her daughter in the terminal phase of viral pneumonia: coughing up blood and gasping for breath (pneumonia kills by slow suffocation). Throughout that last night, according to nurses, she cradled her daughter, kissing and caressing her, whispering endearments; such love, one hopes, would have allayed some of the little girl's terror and suffering. (The accounts were especially poignant to me as they eerily recalled my mother's recollection—she was eight in 1918—of the death of her toddler brother in the arms of her stepmother.)

The hospital listed Sakuntala's cause of death as "dengue fever" and she was cremated before anyone could take a tissue sample. At the funeral, Pranee complained of muscle aches and acute exhaustion, and her family took her to the same clinic that had misdiagnosed her daughter's critical illness as a cold. In a dreadful repeat of the earlier incompetence, Pranee was reassured that she was just suffering from grief and exhaustion. She returned to her factory job, but she soon collapsed and was rushed to a hospital where she died on 20 September, two weeks after her daughter. She was only twenty-six years old.

While public health officials awaited an autopsy report on Pranee, her sister, Pranom, was in medical isolation with similar symptoms. Fortunately, the doctors now suspected bird flu and quickly administered a course of oseltamivir (Tamiflu), a powerful antiviral that, if administered promptly, has proven uniquely effective against the most deadly strains of influenza. While Pranom was recovering, teams of men wearing gas masks and white biosafety suits nervously entered Ban Srisomboon, now a "red zone," to kill, bag, and bury all the remaining birds. Other crews in rubber boots and rain gear sprayed disinfectant on "everything from pickup trucks full of schoolboys to three-wheeled tractors." In an atmosphere of near panic, villagers avoided their neighbors but, at the first sign of a cough or sniffles, raced into the district hospital emergency room, terrified that they had the bird plague. Others implored local monks to exorcise the malevolent spirit that, Stephen King–like, had descended upon their peaceful village.

Their fears were not irrational: on 28 September, WHO announced that Pranee had probably contracted her infection directly from Sakuntala, thus marking the first person-to-person transmission of avian flu since the emergence of the current virulent subtype in 1997. Although the WHO and the Thai government tried to downplay the significance of Pranee's death—"a viral dead end" in the words of one official—influenza researchers knew that the disclosure deserved the headlines and alarm it generated around the world. If the avian virus had acquired enabling genes from a human influenza strain, then Pranee might be only the first of millions of new victims of a plague that in its current incarnation (poultry-to-human transmissions) was killing two-thirds of those it infected.

In this case, the virus was found to be unmodified, suggesting that Pranee had contracted it only because of sustained intimate contact with her daughter's body fluids. But, as the lead researchers pointed out, "this should not be a rationale for complacency"; "the person-to-person transmission of one of the most lethal human pathogens in the modern world should serve as a reminder of the urgent need to prepare for a future influenza pandemic."[5]

The essence of the avian flu threat, as we shall see, is that a mutant influenza of nightmarish virulence—evolved and now entrenched in ecological niches recently created by global agro-capitalism—is searching for the new gene or two that will enable it to travel at pandemic velocity through a densely urbanized and mostly poor humanity. This is a destiny, moreover, that we have largely forced upon influenza. Human-induced environmental shocks—overseas tourism, wetland destruction, a corporate "Livestock Revolution," and Third World urbanization with the attendant growth of megaslums—are responsible for turning influenza's extraordinary Darwinian mutability into one of the most dangerous biological forces on our besieged planet. Likewise, our terrifying vulnerability to this and other emergent diseases has been shaped by concentrated urban poverty, the neglect of vaccine development by a pharmaceutical industry that finds infectious diseases "unprofitable," and the deterioration, even collapse, of public-health infrastructures in some rich as well as poor countries. The evil that visited Ban Srisomboon, in other words, was not some ancient plague awakened from dormancy, if such can exist independent of historical circumstance, but a new form in whose creation we have inadvertently but decisively intervened. And that, as the villagers in Ban Srisomboon avowed, is surely a "sign."

1

Evolution's Fast Lane

*In essence, it's a destructive form of molecular
burglary; flu gets into the building, cracks the
safe, takes what it wants; and wrecks the place
on its way out.*[6]

Pete Davies

The most ferocious of man-eaters is an innocuous companion
of wild ducks and other waterfowl. At the end of every summer, as millions of ducks and geese mass in Canadian and Siberian lakes for their annual migration, influenza blooms. As
researchers first discovered in 1974, the virus replicates harm-
lessly but vigorously in the intestinal tracts of juvenile birds and
is copiously excreted into the water.[7] Other birds ingest this viral soup until as many as one-third of the young ducks and geese
are producing influenza. In northern lakes, moreover, diverse
strains of influenza coexist in the same population, even within
an individual duck; one study in Alberta found twenty-seven
different subtypes in a community of mallards, pintails, and
bluewinged teals.[8]

During their migrations to the Gulf Coast and southern
China, the birds continue to shed virus in their feces for as long as
one month, increasing the likelihood of the infection spreading to

other species of wild and domestic birds. By late fall, however, duck influenza fades to invisibility. Some virologists believe that enough smoldering infection survives in the birds to be rekindled the following August. Others surmise that influenza is tough enough to survive winter under lake ice. In any event, ducks and influenza both return to the same lakes year after year. The cycle, in fact, may be hundreds of thousands, perhaps millions, of years old. In the opinion of one textbook, it is "a classical example of an optimally adapted system."[9] Influenza prospers while ducks remain otherwise unharmed.

Influenza in humans, pigs, and other mammals, on the other hand, is far from such a happy equilibrium; indeed, it is a radically different system of host–parasite interaction due to a variety of factors. In the first place, the virus usually infects the respiratory tract rather than the gut and spreads by an aerosol rather fecal–oral route. Second, it is highly pathogenic, causing an acute respiratory infection that sometimes kills the host. Third, in contrast to genetically stable wild-duck influenzas, the species-jumping versions are extraordinary shape-shifters that constantly alter their genomes to foil the powerful immune systems of human and mammalian hosts. The pandemic threat stems especially from this capacity for ultrafast evolutionary adaptation.

Influenzas are classified into three major genera: A, B, and C. Influenzas B and C have been domesticated by long circulation in human populations. "Genetic studies," a leading expert explains, "suggest that [they] . . . diverged from the avian influenza A viruses many centuries ago."[10] Influenza C is a cause of the so-called common cold, while B produces a classic winter flu, especially among children. Neither is a pandemic threat, although B is responsible for some of the annual influenza mortality in susceptible populations. Influenza A, on the other hand, is still wild and very dangerous. Although its primary reservoir remains among ducks and waterfowl, it is in the early stages of crossing over to humans and other bird and mammal species. Compared to other human pathogens, it is also evolving at record-breaking speed; from year to year its proteins change amino acids to create modified strains requiring new vaccines, a process called *antigenic drift*. Moreover, every human generation or so, a bird or pig version of influenza A will swap genes with a human type of influenza, or more drastically, acquire mutations that permit it to vault over the species barrier. This revolutionary event is called *antigenic shift*, and it signals the imminence of a pandemic. In effect, influenza A reinvents itself as a new disease against which we have no protective immunological memory. In epidemiological parlance (and in contrast to more stable viruses like smallpox), it is a "constantly emerging disease."[11]

To appreciate the true genius of influenza A, it is necessary to know a little about its macromolecules and their stunning evolutionary capabilities. Like all viruses, influenza is a parasitic genome traveling in the company of clever proteins. Under an electron microscope it is revealed to be a spheroid bristling with tiny spikes and mushrooms, rather like an infinitesimal dandelion. The spikes consist of three intertwined molecules of hemagglutinin, an amazing protein that derives its name from its ability to agglutinate red blood cells. The square-headed mushrooms, fewer in number, are powerful enzymes known as neuraminidase. The outer surface of the virus also has a few M2 proteins that function as proton pumps; these allow the virus to adjust the relative acidity of its interior. Inside the virus's lipid jacket—stolen

X

from a host cell—is its strange genome. All living cells, of course, are programmed by the instructions contained in their DNA double helices. Influenza's genetic software, however, consists of single-stranded RNA packaged in eight separate segments known as ribonucleoprotein complexes (RNPs). Inside each of these complexes, an RNA molecule is coiled tightly around a nucleoprotein and bound together with the polymerases required for its synthesis. Inside the host, the virus also produces a nonstructural protein (NS1) which interferes with the cellular interferon-based immune response. Finally, a matrix protein called M1 fills the remaining space, cushioning the RNPs like so much styrofoam popcorn.

This highly competent little assembly is chemically inert until the hemagglutinin spikes make contact with appropriate receptors (actually sialic acid residues) on the surface of certain cells. While hemagglutinin (hence: HA) is the molecular key that influenza uses to unlock and enter host cells, different key configurations are needed to open different cells. Avian influenza HA, for example, generally only unlocks the intestinal cells of waterfowl, while human HA has been refashioned to break into cells in the mucous lining of the respiratory system. This difference in lock and key configurations is generally considered to be the species barrier that prevents avian influenzas from easily circulating among mammals. Recent research has shown, however, that slight amino substitutions in avian HA—perhaps even the change of a single glutamine to leucine—may suffice to unlock human cells.[12]

Once influenza's HA has docked with a host cell, actual entry requires that the big HA molecule be cleaved down the middle to expose key amino acid complexes; some virologists

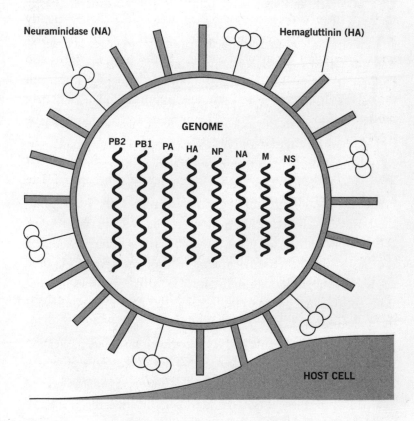

Neuraminidase (NA)

Hemagluttinin (HA)

GENOME

PB2 PB1 PA HA NP NA M NS

HOST CELL

Figure 1   The Influenza Virus

compare this to opening a Swiss army knife. This cleavage is catalyzed by proteases, protein-hungry enzymes in the host organism. Most influenza HAs are fussy in choosing proteases, but some are more promiscuous. The latter probably have faster rates of attack and are correspondingly more virulent. In any case, HA's success at breaking and entering is the *sine qua non* of an influenza infection, and it is the primary target (or *antigen*) of immune response and vaccination. Pandemic influenza is usually defined as the emergence or reappearance of an HA subtype against which most people have no prior immunity.

After HA turns the lock, the influenza virus enters the host cell clothed in some of the host's own plasma membrane. The M2 channel protein then pumps ions into the interior of this capsule (*endosome*). The increased acidity dissolves the membrane and releases influenza's genome segments (the RNPs) into the host cell. The RNPs then flock to the nucleus, where viral RNA replication takes place. Like all viruses, influenza hijacks the host's biosynthetic machinery to produce several hundred copies of itself; in human influenza, the virus also issues instructions to stop making the proteins that the host cell requires for its own survival.

The complex details of RNA transcription and replication are best left to a good virology textbook, but two general aspects of influenza's reproduction are key to understanding its success as a pathogen. First, RNA synthesis is radically error prone. All cellular life (as well as some viruses) depends upon the scrupulous accuracy of DNA polymerase in duplicating genetic information; like an obsessive scholar, it proofreads and corrects every copy of DNA, and the resulting error rate (in bacteria and humans) is thus less than one mistake in every billion nucleotides copied. RNA polymerases, on the other hand, are careless hacks who do not proof or correct their copy. As a result, the error rates in influenza and some other RNA viruses are 1 million times greater than in DNA-based genomes. Each new strand of RNA is a mutant, differing on average from its parental template by at least one nucleotide. (Its progeny are often characterized as a "mutant swarm" or "quasi species" because of their extreme variability.) Influenza, in fact, lives at the very edge of what evolutionary biologists call "error catastrophe." If the error rate were any higher, information integrity would be lost, and the genome would decay into utter gibberish.[13]

To aficionados of complexity theory, then, influenza is an outstanding example of a self-organized system on the edge of chaos.* Such perilous fine-tuning is supposed to optimize complexity and enhance evolutionary fitness, but for what purpose? In wild ducks, genetic hypervariability has seemingly lost its *raison d'être*; older strains of influenza find it easy to earn a living, and different subtypes can coexist peacefully with another. Evolution, according to Robert Webster and William Bean, has resulted in stasis as "the long-term survival of the avian viruses appears to favor those that have not changed, and selection is primarily negative."[14] In humans and other secondary hosts, however, influenza comes under ferocious attack from sophisticated immune systems. This generates intense selective pressure, which in turn kicks evolution into fast forward. "The molecular clocks

---

* Some scientists find influenza's sudden mutations and dramatic shifts too extreme to accept as mere results of RNA genetics. Most famously, the astrophysicist Sir Fred Hoyle and his associate Chandra Wickramasinghe have proposed an extravagant theory positing that influenza is literally extraterrestrial; that it episodically hitchhikes to earth on cosmic dust particles scattered in the tail of comets.

of RNA viruses," writes evolutionary biologist John Holland, "can spin at blinding speeds as compared to those of their hosts." Indeed, their rates of evolution "proceed up to millions-fold faster than that of their hosts."[15]

Influenza A's extraordinary heterogeneity thus becomes a resource for resisting the immune-system onslaught. As rapidly as antibodies defeat one influenza strain, others, more resistant, emerge to take its place—a single amino acid substitution can suffice to thwart an antibody attack. This irresistible drift of influenza's antigenic characteristics ensures its survival in the face of the antibody blitz. Indeed, according to leading researchers, "it may be that human influenza A is unique in that it is able to produce a series of antigenically selected mutants that are as fit as the parental population and is the only virus that undergoes true antigenic drift."[16] Yet if these point mutations ensure influenza viability as a disease from season to season, they do not totally outwit immunological memory. "[T]he high level of partial immunity remaining in the community," Dorothy Crawford explains, "ensures that antigenic drift will not cause a pandemic."[17]

The influenza genome, however, has a second, even more extraordinary, trick up its sleeve: because its RNA is packaged in separate segments, a co-infection of a host cell by two different subtypes of influenza can result in a *reassortment* of their constituent genes. Under the right circumstances, influenzas can trade replicating RNPs like kids swap baseball cards, with the resulting hybrids having gene segments from different parents. Thus the pandemic Asian flu of 1957 contained three avian segments (including a novel HA) along with five RNPs from the previously circulating human subtype. Likewise, the pandemic Hong Kong subtype of 1968 retained six segments of the 1957 genome while adding new avian genes for HA and one of the polymerases. In both cases, the *reassortants* combined avian surface proteins with human-adapted internal proteins; this enabled them to overcome what Taubenberger and Reid characterize as "the twin challenges of being 'new' to its host, while being supremely well adapted to it."[18]

But, given the species barrier raised by HA specificity, how do co-infections of avian and human viruses ever occur? Until the 1997 outbreak, it was generally believed that antigenic shift required the intermediary of pigs: "[F]or influenza viruses, the species barrier to pigs is relatively low when compared with the barrier between birds and humans."[19] Cells in the respiratory systems of swine have the right receptors for both avian and human HA and thus can contract diverse subtypes of influenza A—they are ideal viral blenders. Their critical role, moreover, is supported by epidemiological history: influenza epidemics and pandemics usually emerge first in southern China (especially in Guangdong and the Pearl River Delta) where huge numbers of pigs, domestic ducks, and wild waterfowl live in traditional ecological intimacy.

It should be stressed, however, that reassortment, like mutational drift, is a scattershot process. As a leading researcher at the National Institutes of Health explains, "the vast majority of reassortants between avian and human (or mammalian) influenza viruses contain a gene . . . or gene constellation that prevents the virus replicating efficiently in primates." Nevertheless, "some 25 percent of the resulting recombinant viruses would still be potentially virulent for humans if one of the two parents is a human influenza virus."[20] On rare occasions, it is also possible for novel influenza subtypes to emerge through *recombination*: the splicing together of parts of genes (coding for the same protein) from different species. In a controversial 2001 article in *Science*, three Australian researchers proposed that the devastating 1918 pandemic was triggered by a recombination event involving the HA gene. The spike head, they argued, derived from a swine lineage, while the stalk was encoded by a human gene. This recombinant hemagglutinin, they suggest, may have had "an unusual tissue specificity, such that it spread from the upper respiratory tract to the lungs."[21] (Later, to make matters more complex, we will examine two other possible mechanisms of pandemic emergence: dormancy and direct species jump.)

Whether or not recombination is part of influenza A's repertoire, few other human pathogens—apart from the HIV retrovirus (world champion at wily mutation) and the chief malaria parasite, *Plasmodium falciparum*, seem so invincible. Yet influenza does have its weak points, as can be seen as we complete our sketch of its progress through a host: next, the progeny viruses must be assembled and then execute their escape from the dying host cell. Although research shows that the M1 protein is probably the "major virus assembly organizer," the complex choreography that produces new viral particles out of the separately replicated gene strands and proteins is incompletely understood.[22] The final assembly takes the form of a budding of the new viruses from the cellular membrane. This is sticky business; the problem is that the strong affinity of the HA molecules for the external neuraminic acid residues—the very property that made viral entry possible—now blocks the exit. Neuraminidase (henceforth: NA) overcomes this dilemma by attacking and removing the neuraminic acid residues—if HA is the burglar, NA is the escape artist. Their complementary roles are so important that virologists classify influenza A subtypes by their specific HA and NA: the formula adapted in 1980 is HxNy. (Please remember this. It will avoid confusion later on when you meet a series of bad characters named H3N2, H9N1, H5N1, and so on.)

However the NA mushrooms are more vulnerable than are the HA spikes to antivirals that imitate neuraminic (sialic) acid residues and plug strategic portals in their three-dimensional structures. The development of powerful neuraminidase inhibitors—zanamivir (Relenza) in 1993 and oseltamivir (Tamiflu) in 1997—has been a major breakthrough in the treatment of annual influenza. More importantly, zanamivir and oseltamivir are the *only* medications that are thus far effective in preventing or moderating the acute onset of avian flu (or, for that matter, lab-made clones of the deadly 1918 strain).[23] Because of the difficulties of administering zanamivir—it requires an inhaler—oral oseltamivir tablets are seen as the only practical alternative for mass prophylaxis. Indeed, until (and if) avian flu vaccines become widely available, oseltamivir, as *Science* points out, "would be the world's only initial defense against a pandemic that could kill millions of people."[24] For several years the world's top influenza experts have been urging a crash program to increase oseltamivir production; it is currently manufactured by Roche in a single factory in Switzerland. An international stockpile could then be set aside for emergency use by the WHO. These warnings, as we shall see later, have largely been ignored, and oseltamivir inventories remain woefully insufficient to meet the pandemic needs of a single American state, much less the entire nation or the rest of the world.

2

The Virulence of Poverty

Our worst nightmare may not be a new one.[25]
Richard Webby and Robert Webster

Influenza is both familiar and unknown. Although easily distinguished from most common colds by a characteristic moderate to high fever and dry cough, influenza A can exhibit an extremely broad range of symptoms (including sore throat, headache, bone aches, conjunctivitis, dizziness, vomiting, and diarrhea) that overlap with numerous other so-called "grippes, catarrhs and colds." The continuing, rampant prescription of antibiotics for influenza is proof of the difficulty that most general practitioners and clinic staff face in distinguishing between viral and bacterial infections. "[I]t is now accepted," writes one world authority, "that influenza is quite protean in its manifestations. Influenza cannot be distinguished readily on clinical grounds from other acute respiratory infections, and during virologically confirmed outbreaks of influenza the proportion of influenzal illnesses confirmed by laboratory tests as being influenza is currently about half."[26]

If diagnosis is often mere guesswork, an accurate census of influenza mortality is almost an impossibility: except during pandemics, influenza is usually only the accessory to murder. By destroying the ciliated epithelial cells that sweep dust and germs out of the respiratory tract, flu encourages superinfection by bacteria. (*Haemophilus influenzae*—widely believed in 1918–19 to be the actual pathogen of the pandemic—is a famous fellow traveler.) A lethal synergy is believed to operate between influenza A and pneumonic bacteria, with *Staphylococcus aureus* and *Strepto coccus pneumoniae* being particularly vicious; thus, bacterial pneumonia is the most common, or at least the most clearly associated cause of influenza deaths. But how to distinguish influenza-related cases from the rest of pneumonia mortality? As Registrar General of England William Farr first realized during an influenza epidemic in 1847, the infection's well-defined seasonality (October to March in the Northern Hemisphere) in temperate countries allows a rough calculation of excess mortality by simple subtraction of the annual average from the winter spike.[27]

Although epidemiologists now use sophisticated regression modeling, influenza mortality is still estimated in North America and Europe as excess annual mortality. Recently, however, it has become evident that the traditional reporting category "pneumonia and influenza" shortchanges influenza's deadly impact. Most of the winter spike in ischemic heart disease, diabetes, and cerebrovascular disease mortality may also result from the impact of the annual flu epidemic; conversely, "influenza vaccination has been associated with large reductions in the risks of primary cardiac arrest, recurrent myocardial infection, cardiac disease and stroke."[28] In a normal year, researchers now believe that influenza kills between 36,000 to 50,000 mostly elderly (and especially poor) Americans, a reality that belies the benign image of flu as nothing more than a winter nuisance.[29] Sadly, an infection that primarily kills infants and old people is not likely to arouse as much concern as a disease that kills young or middle-aged adults.

As difficult as it is to estimate flu mortality in this country, global influenza mortality is mere conjecture. "There is," writes one research team, "an under-appreciation and an under-estimation of the impact of influenza in the developing world."[30] It is sometimes said that flu kills 1 million people worldwide each year, but the toll could be considerably higher because annual influenza is the least recognized of all so-called "captains of death." Neither China nor India, for instance, reports flu statistics to the World Health Organization.[31] In tropical countries, moreover, the absence of well-defined seasonality in the incidence of influenza makes estimation of excess mortality difficult. This dearth of data, in turn, has reinforced the stereotype that there is no significant influenza burden in Asia or Africa.

While high death rates from acute respiratory infections in the tropics are often attributed to tuberculosis, recent research has established that a majority of acute respiratory deaths are caused by viruses, and that tropical countries have influenza mortality rates at least equivalent to those in the mid-latitudes. Indeed, "infection probably has an even greater relative impact on the health of persons from developing countries who are already susceptible to complications because of underlying malnutrition, tropical diseases and HIV."[32] As studies in Southeast Asia have shown, "overall influenza-associated mortality in a region with a warm climate, such as Hong Kong, is comparable with that documented in temperate regions." Moreover, infant mortality from influenza is probably considerably higher in low-income tropical countries.[33]

Influenza is most of all a mystery disease in sub-Saharan

Africa. The region is the weakest link in the global influenza-surveillance network coordinated by the WHO: in recent years Côte d'Ivoire, Zambia, and Zimbabwe have closed down their national flu surveillance systems after pleading debt and bankruptcy; currently only South Africa and Senegal actively track flu cases and have the laboratory resources to isolate and characterize subtypes. In the rest of Africa, serious flu cases are commonly conflated with malaria or just added to the "acute respiratory infection" (ARI) grab bag. Yet annual influenza in Africa does often produce explosive local outbreaks, such as the 2002 epidemic in Madagascar which overwhelmed the country's health-care system, or the massive irruption six months later in the Equateur Province of the Democratic Republic of the Congo which yielded shocking rates of secondary pneumonia.[34]

Third World influenza is also largely invisible or poorly studied in the historical record. The apocalyptic pandemic of 1918–19—according to the WHO, "the most deadly disease event in the history of humanity"—is the template for the public-health community's worst fears about the imminent threat of avian influenza.[35] After two generations of cultural amnesia, popular interest in the history and legacy of the "Spanish flu" (so called because uncensored newspapers in neutral Spain were the first to report its arrival) has undergone a dramatic revival in recent years. Since 1974, when Richard Collier published an anecdotal history based on interviews with hundreds of survivors, an impressive succession of historians and science journalists—including Alfred Crosby, Gina Kolata, Pete Davies, and, most recently, John M. Barry—has focused on the far-reaching impacts of the pandemic on American life, medical research, and the outcome of World War I. Several writers have also chronicled the recent expeditions to Alaska and Spitzbergen in the Arctic to try to retrieve the 1918 virus from the frozen cadavers of its victims, as well as the dramatic successes of U.S. Army scientists, led by Jeffrey Taubenberger, in reconstructing much of the 1918 virus's genome.

The threat of a new pandemic, meanwhile, spurs continuing research into many aspects of the 1918 virus's molecular structure; the enigmatic circumstances of its emergence (reassortment or recombination?), its geographical origin (a Kansas army base, the trenches in France, and southern China are all proposed epicenters),[36] and its distinctive mode of attack (which produced singularly high mortality among young adults). Despite renewed scholarly investigation into the 1918 pandemic, however, shockingly little attention has been paid to the disease's ecology in its major theater of mortality in 1918–19: British India. This oversight is analogous to the history of the First World War having been written with a vivid, sustained focus on the campaigns in the Balkans and Gallipoli while devoting only an occasional aside or footnote to the slaughter on the Western Front.

The enormity of influenza's impact on India has never been questioned. For decades the authoritative guide to worldwide pandemic mortality was the 1927 American Medical Association–sponsored study—*Epidemic Influenza*—by Edwin Oakes Jordan, editor of the prestigious *Journal of Infectious Disease*, who had spent years poring over death statistics. The huge spike in mortality during the fall of 1918—U.S. life expectancy fell by ten years—allowed him to make estimates of the pandemic toll despite the absence of influenza data per se (see Table 2.1). Jordan believed that global mortality from influenza was in the range of 20 to 22 million (about 1 percent of the human race), with India alone

Table 2.1.
Pandemic Mortality 1918–19—Revised[37]

Worldwide	(a) 21.64 million	(b) 48.8 to 100 million
Asia	15.78	26 to 36
India	*12.50*	*18.5*
China	. . . . . .	4 to 9.5
East Indies	.80	1.5
Europe	2.16	2.3
Africa	1.35	2.38
W. Hem.	1.40	1.54
USA	.55	.68

(a) Jordan (1927) (b) Johnson & Mueller (2002)

suffering 12.5 million deaths, almost 60 percent of the total. (U.S. flu deaths, by contrast, constituted only 3 percent of the world total.) But at an international conference on the history of the great pandemic, held at University of Cape Town in September 2001, medical demographers Niall Johnson and Juergen Mueller challenged Jordan's estimates "as almost ludicrously low." Reviewing modern research, they came to the conclusion that "global mortality from the influenza pandemic appears to have been of the order of 50 million." Moreover, the two warned that "even this vast figure may be substantially lower than the real toll, perhaps, as much as 100 percent understated." In other words, it is possible that mortality was actually closer to 100 million or more than 5 percent of the contemporary world population. In their revision, Indian deaths (mainly in the deadly second wave of influenza after September 1918) are reckoned at 18.5

million, although another scholar thinks 20 million is more likely.[38]

What explains the extraordinary mortality in India? "Famine and pandemic," observes I. Mills, "formed a set of mutually exacerbating catastrophes." Indeed, these two factors were exquisitely synchronized during the fall of 1918. As Mills explains in one of the few scholarly articles on the Indian experience, the milder first wave of the pandemic arrived in Bombay in June (via the crew of a troop transport) just as the southwestern monsoon was failing throughout much of western and central India; the resulting drought led to soaring grain prices and famine conditions in Bombay, the Deccan, Gujarat, Berar, and, especially, the Central and United Provinces. (Although not mentioned by Mills, grain exports to England and wartime requisitioning practices undoubtedly contributed to price inflation and food shortages as well.) In September, as the famine was worsening, the second— more deadly—wave of influenza arrived, again via Bombay.[39]

What followed was the kind of chain reaction (or positive feedback of disasters) that has become so familiar in the history of the modern Third World. "In Bombay Presidency," writes Mills, "the severe second [influenza] wave came at the time of the harvest of the early crop, and sowing of the late crop. With morbidity estimated to be in excess of 50 percent of the population, and with the concentration of severe attacks in the most productive age range, 20–40 [years], the effect on agricultural production was extreme." The area of grain production decreased by one-fifth while staple food prices doubled.[40] The "absolute lack of any public health organization redoubled infection's impact upon the famished population." The Raj heavily taxed the peasantry to support the Indian Army but spent virtually nothing on rural medicine. ("The Surgeon-General conceded that mortality would have been reduced had it been possible to provide immediate medical aid and suitable nourishment to those attacked.")[41] The American missionary Samuel Higginbottom, who was director of agriculture in the state of Gwalior, wrote to a friend that "influenza has been fearful. Hundreds of bodies daily floating in the river. No official figures have been published for India as a whole, but in villages in Gwalior State that are under my charge the death rate during October and November was from 20 to 60 percent. Cholera, plague, and other epidemics from which India suffers have never shown such a death rate as Influenza."[42]

Desperate refugees from the countryside flooded into the slum districts of Bombay and other cities; there, influenza cut them down by the tens of thousands, "like rats without succour," according to the nationalist paper *Young India*.[43] Mortality, Mills emphasizes, was strictly "class oriented," with almost eight times as many deaths among low-caste people in Bombay as among Europeans or wealthy Indians—the poor seemed to have been the victims of a sinister synergy between malnutrition, which suppressed their immune response to infection, and rampant bacterial pneumonia.[44] Outside of the crowded urban slums, flu mortality was generally highest in the famished west of India rather than in the east, where the crops had not failed.

Presumably hunger played a similar role in influenza mortality in China, the East Indies, and even Germany, where the Allied blockade had reduced the caloric intake of the urban poor, especially women and children, to dangerous levels. Certainly, every writer on the pandemic has noted its particular affinity for poverty, substandard housing, and inadequate diets. The slum districts of port cities, from Boston to Bombay, seemed to offer especially favorable conditions for spread of the pandemic in its more virulent form.[45]

The pandemic also formed lucrative partnerships with other epidemic diseases. Iran was a grim case in point: according to a careful study by historian Amir Afkhami, the nation of 11 million suffered the greatest relative mortality of any major country, between 8 and 22 percent of the total population. The pandemic hitchhiked the military supply route from Bombay to the British occupation force in this supposedly neutral country. Iran was already reeling from several years of drought, famine, cholera outbreaks, and the depredations of marauding armies. In addition, the British had callously aggravated the famine by requisitioning the grain surplus from the large estates, leaving little for a hungry population. Writes Afkhami,

> At the dawn of influenza's outbreak in Iran in the spring of 1918, grain supplies were at a low point, and prices had already more than doubled from the preceding six months (when they had reached a ten-year peak). This scarcity continued even following the spring harvest, and villagers, especially in the southern and central provinces, were scarcely surviving on millet-meal and berries. . . . As if starvation were not enough, in 1918 the Iranian people also had to grapple with a widespread typhus epidemic, which was taking its toll in both urban and rural areas. Consequently, the flu came into an environment already beset by the calamities of war, famine and disease.[46]

But Akfhami argues that the principal multiplier of influenza mortality in Iran, even more than hunger, was malaria. He finds dramatic correlations between malaria incidence and influenza mortality, both among the local population and the Indian troops of the British Army. Cities with chronic malaria, such as Mashhad, had influenza death rates triple those of cities with low malaria rates, such as Tehran. The climax of pandemic mortality in November coincided with the usual "peak period of malignant tertian malarial fevers among Iranians." Akfhami also observes that malaria sufferers, including both Iranians and Indians, were afflicted with anemia and were notoriously susceptible to pulmonary infections.[47]

Poverty, malnutrition, chronic illness, and co-infection were thus powerful determinants of the precise tax that the 1918 influenza exacted from different populations. Indeed, the global pandemic itself was really a constellation of individual epidemics, each shaped by local socioeconomic and public-health conditions. In some countries, such as India and Iran, the co-factors (hunger, malaria, anemia) formed deadly nonlinear synergies with influenza and its secondary infections. Although most of the literature on the 1918 pandemic has focused on its unusual preference for young adults, including the robust and well-fed young soldiers of the American Expeditionary Force in France, the correlation between social class and lethality in virtually every country was no less striking. In the most sophisticated analysis of pandemic mortality yet undertaken—a case-study of the 1918 virus in Sydney—Kevin Cracken and Peter Curson found that "the working class and blue-collar workers experienced the heaviest death rates," particularly in the inner city, and that unemployment was as consistent a predictor of mortality as more conventional epidemiological factors such as persons per room density.[48]

3

The Wrong Lessons

The projections are that this virus will kill one
million Americans in 1976.[49]

HEW Secretary David Mathews

The writer John Barry has characterized the 1918 pandemic as the "first great collision between nature and modern science."[50] Certainly it was a supreme test of the self-confidence that scientific medicine had acquired in the generation following the epochal discoveries of Pasteur and Koch. Many of history's great killers—cholera, rabies, typhoid, anthrax, diphtheria, tuberculosis, even plague—had been successfully unmasked as species of bacteria; and although no one had yet seen one, viruses had been recognized in concept as the cause of polio and other diseases. In the Caribbean U.S. Army doctors had driven back the legendary scourge of yellow fever. Potent vaccines and antitoxins had been developed, and biochemistry had taken giant steps; and in the great hospitals and laboratories of Berlin, London, Paris, New York, and Baltimore, all the foundations seemingly had been laid for the defeat of infectious disease.

In addition, World War I mobilized an unprecedented medical effort. As Barry emphasizes, the world's top researchers all anticipated that the Great War would unleash a major epidemic of some kind. But no one anticipated that it would be influenza; indeed, before 1918 flu was not considered a serious killer. Global outbreaks in 1889 and 1898 had, to be sure, raised mortality, but scarcely on the scale of the bubonic plague pandemic of 1894–1918 which ultimately killed millions and briefly threatened to cause the collapse of world commerce. Under grim wartime conditions, with millions of soldiers mired in the mud and filth of trench warfare or overcrowded in squalid hospitals and training camps, pneumonia was a grave danger, but influenza was considered to be merely one of its several causes, along with measles.

In the winter of 1916–17, the British Army experienced a vexing outbreak of acute pneumonia that was accompanied by heliotrope cyanosis—the victims' faces turned blue as their lungs drowned in blood—at its huge encampment at Etaples in France. British researchers have recently proposed that this incident was the first "seeding" of the influenza subtype that became pandemic in the summer of 1918. Army doctors at the time, however, diagnosed the outbreak as epidemic bronchitis and were shocked when the same terrifying symptoms returned on an epic scale with clearly identifiable influenza eighteen months later.[51]

Barry's much-praised book, *The Great Influenza*, provides a gripping account of the desperate campaign mounted by America's leading pulmonary specialists and epidemiologists to contain the disease as the new plague sowed death and panic in the early fall of 1918. Like their European counterparts, they never came close to identifying the true pathogen or creating an effective vaccine, so in the end, public-health officials everywhere fought influenza with the same ancient weapons that Renaissance city-states had used to resist bubonic plague: quarantines and face masks. In a few exceptional cases—American Samoa and Australia—draconian quarantines excluded the pandemic or at least delayed its arrival until its virulence had subsided. Elsewhere the influenza firestorm raged on until it had simply burnt up all available human fuel. With some 500 million people estimated to have been infected, the pandemic was modern medicine's greatest defeat.

But science does not celebrate defeat. Because the self-image of twentieth-century medicine is organized around a heroic mythology of progressive victory against disease, the 1918 catastrophe—that "great shadow cast upon the medical profession"—was quickly repressed in popular memory.[52] After a final flare-up of virulence in winter 1919, the pandemic died away, and influenza research then lost its global urgency. Unlike previous plagues that had laid siege to society for years or decades on end, the great influenza—in essence, a viral atomic bomb—did most of its killing in a single season. Many at the time thought (and some still think today) that it was an unrepeatable aberration, part of the larger nightmare ecology of 1914–18. The pandemic's mystery persisted, however, and a small but committed cadre of microbiologists soldiered on in their laboratories. By the late 1920s they had discarded the once-orthodox belief in a bacterial pathogen and had begun to look for an influenza virus. A swine variety was isolated in 1930 and, using ferrets as surrogates, its human counterpart was identified during a London flu epidemic three years later; both were believed to be offspring of the 1918 killer, with today's opinion favoring the idea that humans passed the virus to pigs, rather than vice-versa.[53]

After Pearl Harbor, Washington again began to worry about

influenza. The senior officers in the surgeon general's office had been young doctors on the frontlines of the 1918 pandemic, and they were haunted by the threat of another pandemic in the barracks. A renowned University of Michigan researcher, Dr. Thomas Francis, who had discovered influenza A's antigenic diversity in 1936 and isolated influenza B in 1940, was appointed head of the Influenza Commission, and his young protégé, Jonas Salk, was charged with carrying out vaccine field trials in 1943. Within a year, a safe and effective experimental vaccine using inactivated viruses grown in fertile eggs was dispelling (forever, some thought) the specter of 1918.[54] However, in the winter of 1946–47, the Francis/Salk vaccine (based on 1934 and 1943 strains) totally failed to provide protection against a new flu. Although the 1947 outbreak (a "pseudo-pandemic") infected hundreds of millions across the globe, it fortunately lacked pandemic lethality; current opinion is that the absence of any cross-immunity between earlier strains and the 1947 flu probably represented an extreme case of mutation within a subtype (H1N1) which otherwise preserved the basic surface antigen (HA and NA) characteristics of 1918.[55]

The 1946–47 failure demonstrated the need to annually update vaccine composition based on careful international screening for newly emergent strains. The new World Health Organization was spurred to establish a world influenza center under the leadership of the famous flu researcher Sir Christopher Andrewes at the British National Institute for Medical Research (NIMR) at Mill Hill, London; this became the cornerstone of today's global influenza surveillance system. Affiliated national laboratories send unknown influenza strains to London (or now, to Atlanta, Melbourne, or Tokyo) for rapid identification. Based on worldwide reports, the WHO laboratories then provide drug manufacturers with candidate strains for the next season's flu vaccine. This system faced its first great test in 1957 when a new flu emerged in the southeastern Chinese province of Yunnan (also the likely origin of the 1894 plague pandemic). Because air travel was still a relatively uncommon mode of transportation, the virus spread by traditional overland routes, via Russia to Europe, and by sea to the Western Hemisphere. Unlike the 1946–47 virus, this was not a mutation of the 1918 strain, but a genuine reassortant—probably arising in pigs—with avian surface proteins (HA and NA) and human-flu internal proteins. H2N2—as it was later classified—was, in other words, a new pandemic influenza.

In the United States, the Eisenhower administration rebuffed appeals from public-health experts for a mass vaccination campaign. Although the surgeon general did appropriate small sums for influenza surveillance, the Republicans in power relied upon free enterprise to develop and distribute the vaccine. "The official national public policy at that time," writes Gerald Pyle, "was that the private sector—[drug producers], physicians and hospitals—could easily deal with the problem."[56] But in the case of influenza, without government coordination classical supply-and-demand relationships work mischievously. The vaccine needs to be produced in quantity for immunization at least a month before the peak of an epidemic, but most of the market demand from individual consumers comes only after the epidemic is in full course. Thus the pharmaceutical industry in fall 1957 was, according to J. Donald Miller and June Osborne, "too little and too late. By mid-October of 1957, when the epidemic reached its peak, less than 30 million doses of influenza vaccine had been fully tested for release, and only 7 million persons had actually received the benefit of immunization."[57]

Fortunately, the Asian flu seldom produced the viral pneumonia, cyanosis, and acute respiratory distress that so gruesomely killed off young adult victims in 1918. An arsenal of powerful new antibiotics, moreover, gave doctors unprecedented control over secondary bacterial infections. Still, 2 million people worldwide were later estimated to have perished in the pandemic, including 80,000 Americans, many of whom might have been saved by timely vaccination.[58] In the opinion of public-health veterans, these deaths were the dismal price of the failure of Eisenhower's reliance upon the invisible hand of private enterprise to do the work of government.[59]

Eleven years later a third pandemic strain was isolated in Hong Kong, although it likely had its origins in neighboring Guangdong. This reassortant, again probably originating inside a pig, conserved the 1957 NA but added a new duck HA (thus becoming H3N2). It was fabulously contagious (500,000 cases in Hong Kong in a few weeks), but unexpectedly mild-mannered, probably because of widespread cross-immunity to its familiar NA. Like an aging rock band on a revival tour, the Hong Kong flu (H3N2) carefully retraced the itinerary of the 1957 Asian flu (H2N2), although its progress was now accelerated by air travel—GIs returning from Vietnam promptly brought it back to California in September 1968. The drug companies again failed to deliver the vaccine in time. "At the peak of the epidemic," write Miller and Osborne, "only 10 million doses of vaccine had been distributed and no more than 6 million individuals had been protected; again, a large store of unused vaccine remained after the epidemic had passed." If H3N2 had been more virulent, a catastrophe might have resulted. About 34,000 Americans died in the event, as did 700,000 others across the world.[60]

The Hong Kong flu left an ambiguous legacy. For many politicians and nonspecialists in the medical community, the relatively mild outcome relaxed apprehensions about pandemic influenza. "[M]any health-policy makers," writes Pyle, "felt no need for an inoculation program."[61] Moreover, the generation of doctors who had experienced the pandemic of 1918 were retiring from research, and new medical school students inherited little more than folklore about hyperlethal influenza strains—and vaccines and antibiotics seemed to be holding an old monster firmly in check. This false sense of security was reinforced by scientific ignorance: despite some important breakthroughs, such as the technique of negative staining that allowed influenza viruses to be photographed under an electron microscope, surprisingly little new ground had been gained in understanding the molecular chemistry of infection or the evolution of the influenza genome. "It was unsuspected [for example] that influenza viruses from animals and birds are involved in the origin of pandemic strains of influenza."[62]

Influenza specialists, however, took away different lessons from the 1957 and 1968 experiences. They were appalled by the unnecessary loss of life and the inefficiency of the profit-driven vaccine marketplace. Pharmaceutical corporations manufactured too little vaccine, and most of it failed to reach such key vulnerable groups like elderly people, pregnant women, and asthmatics. "In 1975, for example," Miller and Osborne write, "less than 20 percent of the group for whom the vaccine was recommended were actually immunized; much of the remaining vaccine had gone to corporations which purchased flu vaccine in bulk and administered it to their young, healthy employees to reduce wintertime attrition due to the flu. The influenza fighters, in contrast, argued for a federally-supported vaccination program for the country's high-risk population, as well as lobbying for a much more timely and aggressive Washington response to the next pandemic.[63]

New discoveries soon supported the case for taking influenza more seriously. After 1968, researchers made a number of dramatic breakthroughs. Virologists, for the first time, were actually able to see the distinctive shapes of the HA and NA molecules. They also confirmed that antigenic drift was the result of point mutation (amino acid substitution) and that HA and NA mutated independently. Even more importantly, they identified genetic reassortment as the probable mechanism for the emergence of new pandemic subtypes; with the parallel discovery of influenza's natural home in ducks and waterfowl, researchers could begin to trace the virus's modern family tree (see Table 3.1). They ultimately identified 15 antigenically distinctive HAs and 9 different NAs in the avian reservoir, for a total of 135 hypothetical subtypes. The evolution of human influenza, it was now clear, was primarily driven by the crossing over of new HA proteins from waterfowl—after its deadly debut, each pandemic form then settled down to earn its living by modest mutation. Blood sera studies of the 1957 and 1968 pandemics, moreover, indicated that elderly people had some immunity to the new pandemic HAs. Researchers, accordingly, postulated that an H2 subtype had caused the 1889 pandemic, and an H3 the 1898 pandemic. Their reemergence in the postwar period was interpreted as evidence that influenza had hiding

Table 3.1.
Influenza A Dynasties

Era	Origin	Subtype	Mode of Antigenic Shift
1890s	Guangdong	H2N2	unknown
1900s	?	H3N8	unknown
1918–57	Kansas (?)	H1N1	species jump or recombination
1957–68	Yunnan	H2N2	reassortment (pig?)
1968–present	Guangdong	H3N2	reassortment (pig?)
1977–present	China or USSR	H1N1	reintroduction from cryptic reservoir
1997	Guangdong	H5N1	species jump

places or cryptic reservoirs where it could slumber for decades, or even generations.[64]

The vistas opened by influenza research in the 1970s were breathtaking, but new knowledge only seemed to deepen the fundamental mysteries. The molecular basis of flu virulence remained unknown, as did the viral component responsible for catastrophic cyanosis. No one could convincingly explain why new subtypes usually extinguished the old, or how seemingly extinct lineages could suddenly reemerge, nor could researchers predict which avian hemagglutinin (an H5 or H7, for example) would next cross the species barrier. Some believed that only a few HAs were endowed with the ability to successfully reassort with human flu genes, while others conjectured that all avian HAs were potential new human influenzas. There was broad agreement, however, that medicine needed to heed influenza's unpredictable evolutionary potential. The revelation of an unexpectedly diverse wild gene pool implied that 1918 might not have been such an aberration after all.

On 13 February 1976, the *New York Times* carried an op-ed piece by Dr. Edwin Kilbourne, a leader of the younger generation of influenza researchers. Kilbourne warned that a new pandemic might be close at hand: "Worldwide epidemics, or pandemics, of influenza have marked the end of every decade since the 1940s—at intervals of exactly eleven years—1946, 1957, 1968. A perhaps simplistic reading of this immediate past tells us that 11 plus 1968 is 1979, and urgently suggests that those concerned with public health had best plan without further delay for an imminent natural disaster." The very same day, communicable-disease officials at the Centers for Disease Control (CDC) in Atlanta were discussing disturbing laboratory findings. New Jersey public health officials had sent the CDC cultures of an unidentified flu that had killed one Army recruit and hospitalized several others at Fort Dix; Dr. Walter Dowdle, the director of CDC's lab, now reported that the mysterious virus was swine flu, a variant of H1N1 that was believed to be genetically closer to the original pandemic strain than the attenuated human genotypes that had circulated from 1920 until they were replaced by H2N2 in 1957. In the worst-case scenario, the great killer of 1918 had been resurrected and posed acute danger to anyone born after 1956 (who thus lacked H1N1 immune memory).[65]

CDC Director David Sencer canvassed the opinions of other experts, but the crucial responsibility for characterizing a pandemic crisis was his. In an emergency meeting with David Mathews, secretary of Health, Education, and Welfare (HEW),

Sencer—supported by his boss, Dr. Theodore Cooper—made the case for universal immunization. Any decision had to be made punctually, for Washington had only a brief window of opportunity to order the vast quantity of fertile eggs required to manufacture a vaccine for the next flu season. Mathews, it turned out, had just finished reading Alfred Crosby's new book, *Epidemic and Peace: 1918,* and he was thus vividly aware of the carnage wrought by the 1918 pandemic. On 15 March, the secretary sent a note to the director of the budget, warning that "the indication is that we will see a return of the 1918 flu virus." Of course, 1976 was an election year, and the White House was stunned when it learned of Mathews's memo. President Gerald Ford, already being pressured by Ronald Reagan's succcess in the early Republican primaries, hardly wanted voters dropping dead of influenza on the way to polling stations in November. Accordingly, he tried to turn the swine flu threat into a political asset by dramatically announcing a crash program to vaccinate more than 100 million Americans.[66]

The administration, however, quickly discovered the vagaries of relying upon the marketplace to supply the emergency vaccine, as well as the difficulties inherent in fragmented local governments supervising mass immunization. Since a 1974 court decision that found drugmaker Wyeth liable for the calamitous side effects of its polio vaccine, the big pharmaceutical companies had been rushing to drop vaccines from their product lines. To induce the companies to start up fertile egg production lines, Ford had to bribe them with $135 million appropriated from Congress for the purchase of vaccines. He then had to submit to blatant extortion by the casualty insurance industry, which refused to provide coverage to the manufacturers unless the federal government agreed to indemnify any claims against the insurers. (An incredulous California congressman, Henry Waxman, asked Theodore Cooper: "Dr. Cooper, are you in effect saying that the insurance industry is using the possibility of a swine flu pandemic as an excuse to blackmail the American people into paying higher insurance rates?") The manufacturing processes, moreover, were proprietary secrets: although the Food and Drug Administration (FDA) had to approve the final vaccines, the government could exert little direct quality control over their production. As a result, Parke-Davis produced several million doses of the wrong strain, and general industry output fell below government expectations.[67]

While the Ford administration was wrestling with these supply-side problems, there was eerie silence on the demand side. The Fort Dix outbreak had died away and no new swine flu cases had emerged on the East Coast or, according to the WHO, anywhere else in the world. One of the CDC's key advisors, polio vaccine pioneer Albert Sabin, counseled Sencer that it would be best to actively stockpile the new vaccine in the public-health network but delay the actual immunization campaign, except for high-risk groups, until swine flu reemerged. Sencer felt that approach was too risky, because air travel now guaranteed that any pandemic would be "jet-spread" within hours. Immunization began in October, with very uneven zeal across the country: some localities, such as Delaware, organized impressive campaigns that resulted in 80 percent coverage, while others, like New York City (where the *Times* editorialized against the program), made only risible gestures resulting in less than 10 percent of the population being immunized. By election eve, with no sign of the dreaded swine flu, public misgivings about the immunization campaign were widespread; two weeks after Jimmy Carter's defeat of Ford, the deaths of several elderly people from the rare Guillain-Barré syndrome were circumstantially linked to the vaccine, and immunization was abruptly halted.[68]

From that point on, swine flu became synonymous with political fiasco. Carter's new HEW secretary, Joseph Califano, asked two Harvard scholars, Richard Neustadt and Harvey Fineberg, to undertake a case-study of the Ford administration's response to the Fort Dix outbreak. Although Neustadt and Fineberg discovered a definite chain of error, including exaggerated estimates of swine flu's similarity to the 1918 virus and the CDC's failure to heed Sabin's advice about stockpiling, they found it impossible to dismiss the CDC's original apprehensions as irrational or irresponsible. Indeed, Califano himself later conceded that he would have probably made the same decision as Mathews, his ill-fated predecessor. As Neustadt and Fineberg document, expert opinion inside the communicable disease community leaned toward the position that overreaction had been preferable to no reaction. (Or, as Edwin Kilbourne put it, "better a vaccine without an epidemic than an epidemic without a vaccine.")[69] On Capitol Hill, however, there was little sympathy for HEW or the CDC.[70]

The most vicious backlash came not from opposition Democrats, but from the Reagan wing of the Republican Party. When the Carter administration tried to fund a permanent federal flu vaccination program in 1978 it ran into fierce opposition from Senator Richard Schweiker of Pennsylvania in the Senate Health Subcommittee. "It is really sort of ironic," the senator scolded Califano. "We just came through the worst medical disaster in history in terms of modern technology, and you want to give them a prize for what has been done." Two years later, Reagan appointed Schweiker as secretary of Health and Human Services (the cabinet successor to HEW) and the program was terminated. Under Reagan and Schweiker federal grants for successful immunization programs for common diseases such as measles were also drastically cut, and influenza vaccine development was handed back to a pharmaceutical industry that had less enthusiasm than ever for the product. The trend—endorsed by Carter and Califano—toward more widespread, even universal, annual flu immunization was stopped cold in its tracks.

Influenza, indeed, became something of a Washington pariah, "the top of no one's list," according to Neustadt and Fineberg.[71] Careers had been wrecked by implosion of the immunization campaign, and no ambitious public-health official wanted to risk the ignominy that Congress had inflicted upon former CDC Director Sencer and his immediate superior, Dr. Cooper. Over succeeding decades, moreover, the swine flu episode has become even more of a black legend militating against proactive public-health initiatives. Even in the late 1990s, with the emergence of the most deadly strain of influenza ever seen by science, the nonepidemic of 1976 was still casting a larger shadow over federal policy-making than the infinitely more serious 1918 pandemic.

4

Birds of Hong Kong

A new phase seems to have begun in the evolution of avian flu viruses. They have found their way directly to man.[72]

Jaap Goudsmit

In April 1997 Hong Kong issued a set of postage stamps celebrating the migratory birds that flock each winter to the city's Deep Bay and the Mai Po marshes. Deep Bay's mangrove swamps are a freshwater/saltwater interface "rich with pickings for birds," while Mai Po, although now surrounded by the skyscraper New Towns of Yuen Long and Tin Shui Wai, is such a luxuriant bird habitat that it has been designated "a wetland of international importance."[73] Hong Kong is proud of preserving so much avian diversity next door to extraordinary urban density. Indeed it is a bird-crazy city: thousands of residents are avid birdwatchers, and Kowloon's famed Bird Garden is one of the world's largest marketplaces for exotic birds of all kinds. In 1997, moreover, the poultry industry was still thriving in the New Territories, supplying ducks, geese, and chickens for sale in the live-poultry markets (also called "wet markets") that are such colorful parts of the urban mosaic. Birds of one kind or another seem to be everywhere.

One of the birds depicted on a new stamp is a handsome,

medium-sized duck called falcated teal. The drakes—somewhat larger than their North American cousins—have dark bills, white throats, and glossy green heads and crests. The teals breed in eastern Siberia before their annual fall migration to the Pearl River Delta and the Mai Po marshes. They like to forage in rice fields or float in freshwater ponds, where they often come into contact with the domestic ducks that are such an integral part of south Chinese agriculture. The teals are treasured for their beautiful plumage and are frequently kept in captivity (again, often alongside domesticated ducks and other birds). Like other wild ducks, they are also safe havens for influenza. Amongst the flu subtypes identified in a Hong Kong teal is H5N1. That might well make the falcated teal the duck of the apocalypse.

In March 1997, a month before the bird stamps were issued, chickens started dying on a farm near Yuen Long and the Mai Po marshes; they displayed the unmistakable violent symptoms of Highly Pathogenic Avian Influenza (HPAI). As Pete Davies explains in his account of the outbreak: "It's an ugly business. The virus spreads through the bloodstream to infect every tissue and organ; the brain, stomach, lungs, and eyes all leak blood in a body-wide hemorrhage until, from the tips of their combs to the claws on their feet, the birds literally melt."[74] The disease spread to two nearby poultry farms, and as is so often the case with HPAI outbreaks, almost all the birds died. The virus was identified by Hong Kong University researchers as H5N1, a subtype first isolated in 1959. Veterinary virologists had seen it on only two other occasions: during a devastating outbreak in Pennsylvania in 1983 that forced authorities to cull 20 million chickens, and, more recently, among English turkeys in 1991.

The gruesome pathology of so-called "fowl plague" was

first described in 1878, but the pathogen was not confirmed as influenza A until 1955. Episodic outbreaks in poultry farms along major migratory flyways in California and Minnesota suggested to scientists that it originated in ducks and other waterfowl. Like all influenza, HPAI is essentially mysterious: it flares up unexpectedly among chickens and turkeys in different countries, continents, and hemispheres. Until recently, it has been relatively rare, with fifteen localized outbreaks between 1959 and its sudden appearance in Hong Kong in 1997. HPAI in all of these instances was caused by influenza subtypes containing either H5 or H7; researchers believe that these hemagglutinins contain extra basic amino acids at their cleavage sites that amplify virulence by allowing viruses to invade a broader variety of tissues and, possibly, species.[75] But there was no evidence at all to suggest that these avian superviruses posed any threat to humans, not even to the poultry workers who tended the ill birds and cleaned up in the aftermath of HPAI's carnage. "In fact," Hong Kong researchers emphasized, "attempts to transmit experimentally a number of avian virus subtypes directly to humans were not successful." The species barrier was believed to be insurmountable.[76]

After agricultural authorities killed off the remaining sick chickens in April, HPAI seemingly disappeared, with extensive testing failing to reveal any further traces of H5N1 in New Territory chicken farms or Hong Kong's live-poultry markets. Veterinary scientists relaxed. Then in mid-May a three-year-old boy—previously in perfect health—was admitted to Queen Elizabeth Hospital in Kowloon with a sore throat, fever, and abdominal pain. Despite top-flight intensive care, his condition deteriorated catastrophically, and he died on 21 May. Physicians and nurses were appalled by the relentless cascade of disasters that wracked his tiny body: viral pneumonia, acute respiratory distress syndrome (ARDS), Reye's syndrome, and finally, kidney and liver failure. The local department of health ran tests on secretions from the dead child's throat and found an unusual influenza subtype that it could not identify; frozen samples were sent off in June to two of WHO's four collaborating centers (CDC in Atlanta and NIMR in London), as well as to the National Influenza Center in Rotterdam.

In retrospect, influenza experts would applaud the vigilance of Hong Kong health officials. The city, with its world-class medical community, is the sentinel for influenza surveillance in the south China region, where interspecies transmission of viral strains is believed to be most frequent and intense. If the three-year-old had died in neighboring Guangdong, or for that matter, in any of the poorer countries of southeast Asia, it is unlikely that the identification of his pathogen would have been pursued with such vigor.[77] The team in Rotterdam was the first to uncover the lethal strain's identity. As Davies recounts, the Dutch worked throughout July in an unsuccessful attempt to match the Hong Kong virus against their reference archive of human and swine influenzas. Baffled by the failure of the virus to react with any of their antisera, in early August they tested it against a long-shot H5N1 reagent that been brought back from the Memphis laboratory of the famous influenza authority Robert Webster. To the consternation of the Rotterdam team, it was a positive match.[78]

The Dutch result was soon confirmed by Atlanta and London, but no one was yet ready to accept that H5N1 had actually vaulted the species barrier and killed the child in Hong Kong. It seemed more plausible that Hong Kong public-health scientists had unwittingly submitted a contaminated sample. Leaving nothing to conjecture, the Dutch, followed by the CDC and WHO, sent experts, including Webster, to double-check conditions in the Hong Kong lab. They soon discovered that the Chinese had been scrupulous in their procedures—there was no contamination. H5N1 was indeed the killer, and as Webster later discovered, it was almost identical to the strain that had killed the chickens in March. A slight hemagglutinin mutation—a difference of only three amino acids—had apparently allowed the bird virus to open the lock on human cells and infect the child.[79]

It was a staggering, paradigm-shifting discovery. This H5N1 was not a reassortant, as textbooks predicted, but an avian virus that had come to roost in the human body with a little help from genetic drift. Having made such a seemingly impossible species leap, moreover, there was no theoretical reason why H5N1 could not subsequently reassort with human flu genes in the lungs of a co-infected human; pigs might not be the virus's indispensable intermediaries after all. A pandemic of frightening lethality therefore might be imminent, and it was desperately important for the team of international flu experts in Hong Kong to uncover the exact circumstances of the child's infection.

The most obvious hypothesis—that he had encountered sick chickens at one of the New Territory farms or in a local live-poultry market—turned out to be unlikely. Indeed, the only plausible avian contact that researchers could establish were some chicks and ducklings that had been pets at his preschool; the baby birds had died mysteriously, but when researchers painstakingly tested dust in the playroom they could find no sign of the virus. On the other hand, extensive blood testing revealed that a handful of the child's contacts, including a playmate, a nurse, and a

few others (but not his immediate family), had antibodies to
H5N1. Five poultry workers also displayed immunological evidence of contact with the virus, but none had become sick.
Meanwhile, the trail grew cold, and no more cases appeared:
perhaps the child's death had been a fluke. The international experts returned home.

Virologists remained unsettled by the fierce behavior of
H5N1/97 in the laboratory. "It reproduced much faster than
ordinary flu strains, and in cells that ordinary flu strains couldn't
live in, and if you grew it in eggs, it killed them. This virus, said
Lim [a Hong Kong scientist], was like an alien." Indeed, when
veterinary researchers in Athens, Georgia, infected a poultry
flock with the recently isolated human strain, the entire flock
died within a day. Horrified scientists, who had never seen such a
rapid killer, immediately donned biohazard containment suits
and dosed themselves with antivirals; this ignited a controversy
about the safety protocols necessary for work with the Hong
Kong virus. Influenza diagnostic labs, at least in the United
States, were not equipped with the elaborate containment systems required for working with such a potent virus: federal
biosafety guidelines had not anticipated an influenza that acted
like the nightmare protagonist of a sci-fi thriller. (Nor did they
foresee the possibility that by 2004 scientists would use reverse
genetic engineering to re-create the 1918 monster in their labs.)
A majority of the research community now decided that H5N1
research should be confined to a small number of Biosafety
Level 3-plus or Level 4 labs, but a few scientists chafed under the
restrictions (and were later accused of cutting corners on safety).
Lurking in the background was the memory of the unexpected
resurrection of the H1N1 virus in 1977, an outbreak that almost

certainly resulted from the inadvertent escape of the strain from a Russian, or possibly Chinese, laboratory. H5N1, however, might be incomparably more dangerous.[80]

None of the journalistic accounts of the 1997 outbreak mention the extreme weather, but it was the wettest year in Hong Kong's meteorological record—a massive Pacific El Niño event brought typhoons and torrential rain to southern China throughout the summer. (Did the deluges wash away the poultry excrement that spread the infection?) The city was still soaked when the pandemic threat suddenly returned at the beginning of winter. A six-year-old with heart problems was hospitalized on 6 November with ordinary flu symptoms; he recovered quickly, but the lab assay confirmed he had H5N1. Two weeks later, a teenager and two adults—all unrelated—were hospitalized with the virus. State-of-the-art intensive care failed to prevent the onset of viral pneumonia or other macabre complications like those that had killed the toddler in May; two of the patients died in December. Meanwhile, flu experts from Atlanta, Memphis, and Tokyo were flying back to Hong Kong. The WHO set up a special Pandemic Task Force and expected the worse.

The city was on the edge of panic. Although Hong Kong had just been returned to Chinese sovereignty, the local press was unfettered in its coverage of the new outbreak. Opposition politicians hammered the administration of Tung Chee-hwa for any perceived hesitancy in its response to the threat.[81] Throughout December public anxiety was reinforced by the seemingly random fashion in which new human cases were appearing across the territory. In addition, the regular flu season had started early, thus increasing the chance of co-infection and reassortment between H5N1 and the prevailing H3N2 human virus. CDC's top scientist on the scene, Dr. Keiji Fukuda, later reminisced to the *New York Times*: "None of us was sleeping much. The adrenaline was really flowing at this point. A pandemic was suddenly not a misty historical possibility. It seemed very current."[82]

Parallels with 1918 were becoming obvious. Like its ancestor, H5N1 was now focusing its virulence on healthy adults. Of the seventeen new cases diagnosed between early November and the end of December, eight children, happily, all recovered, with few complications; five of the nine teenage and adult victims, however, were destroyed by viral pneumonia and ARDS. The silver lining (and scientific paradox) was that the virus's success in replicating so efficiently inside humans was not yet matched by equivalent transmissibility. The pandemic spark existed, but there was not yet any conflagration. Nonetheless, frantic Hong Kong authorities bought up a large share of the available world supply of the antiviral medication rimantadine as a precaution.

Then in mid-December the "missing link in the epidemiology of avian influenza" suddenly revealed itself: chickens started dropping dead on poultry farms and in the city's markets. The poultry epidemic that had vanished in the spring was now everywhere: H5N1 infected at least 20 percent of the city's chickens, as well as a few domestic ducks and geese. (Not surprisingly, other influenza A subtypes with H9, H6, and H11 hemagglutinins were also identified in birds, although none was yet a homicide suspect.) The virus load in the city's birds seemed to be approaching some kind of ominous critical mass, but there was no precedent for understanding the consequences of such a large-scale animal epidemic in the heart of a great city. Public-health workers, however, did establish that most of the sick humans had had direct contact with poultry, which made it less likely that H5N1 had succeeded in passing from person to person.[83] On the other hand, some of the infected poultry had come from Guangdong and scientists worried that a stealth epidemic—either undiagnosed or concealed for political reasons—already existed in other parts of the Pearl River Delta. (Evidence later would emerge of an epidemic among geese in Guangdong the previous year.)

Hong Kong's local government could not make public-health decisions for the rest of China, but it acted decisively to protect its own citizens. Warned by scientists that there was not a second to lose, on 27 December authorities ordered the destruction of all 1.6 million live poultry within the city and its environs; they also embargoed the import of live birds from Guangdong and disinfected the city's markets. The bird cull, as agriculture official Clive Lau explained to reporters from *Asia-Week*, was a dismal business:

> One evening, Lau was at the command center and phoned a four-person team on a farm with 20,000 chickens. In four hours they had killed 35. The unpenned birds were proving remarkably elusive. "You start killing and killing and killing," says Lau. "And there are still thousands of birds." Often the reluctant butchers had to break necks and slit throats. The birds struggled and scratched. Some people threw up from the smell. Others broke down and cried.
>
> Lau is father to a one-year-old boy and five-year-old girl. All the while, he fretted that he could catch the virus and pass it to them. Back home, the first thing he did was shout, "Get away from me!" He threw his

bloody shoes outside, stripped to his underwear and ran to the bathroom, yelling at his family not to come near. After cleaning up, throwing away his clothes and scrubbing his shoes, Lau at last said hello to his children. He wanted to kiss them, but didn't dare.[84]

Other Hong Kong residents were no less apprehensive. The day before the slaughter, a Filipina domestic worker was diagnosed with bird flu, and the whole city worried whom would be next—every sneeze, cough, and fever that winter was a source of anxiety. Day after day, week after week, health workers nervously tested and retested every case of serious influenza or respiratory distress. Apart from the domestic worker who died in mid-January, they found no further trace of H5N1, and so the economic crisis in Southeast Asia began to displace flu from the headlines again. Authorities very cautiously allowed the sale of live chickens and other terrestrial poultry to resume, although live ducks and geese were banned; in addition, all poultry imported from Guangdong was now screened for influenza.

City authorities celebrated a victory although researchers knew that "an H5N1 pandemic had been averted rather than prevented." A trio of Hong Kong microbiologists who had been at the eye of the storm—Yi Guan, Malik Peiris, and Ken Shortridge—wrote that "the H5N1/97 virus was possibly one or two mutational events from achieving pandemicity." These researchers also began to unravel the virus's genealogy. They found evidence that aquatic bird influenzas had reassorted themselves within the mixing vessel of a quail before jumping to chickens. The two water birds were likely a goose, and yes, possibly a teal.[85]

5

A Messy Story

An outbreak, like a story, should have a coherent plot.[86]

Philip Mortimer

In 1993 Oxford University Press published a collection of essays, edited by Rockefeller University's Stephen Morse, on new and reemergent viruses. Unlike most scholarly anthologies, Morse's volume combined the indisputable authority of the field's leading researchers (including influenza's "emperor" and "pope," respectively, Edwin Kilbourne and Robert Webster) with an unusual sense of urgency. Written in the shadow of the AIDS pandemic and the Ebola outbreak in Africa, *Emerging Viruses* warned that global economic and environmental change were speeding the evolution and interspecies transmission of new viruses, some of which might be as deadly as HIV. In his foreword, Richard Krause of the National Institutes of Health pointed to the new ecologies of disease resulting from globalization. "Microbes thrive in these 'undercurrents of opportunity' that arise through social economic change, changes in human behavior, and catastrophic events. . . . They may fan a minor outbreak into a widespread epidemic."[87]

One such catastrophic event is Third World urbanization,

which is shifting the burden of global poverty from the countrysides to the slum peripheries of new megacities. Ninety-five percent of future world population growth will be in the poor cities of the South, with immense consequences for the ecology of disease. This concentration of the world population in deprived conditions, more than global population growth per se, undergirds what William McNeill calls the "Law of the Conservation of Catastrophe."[88]

McNeill is a well-known University of Chicago historian of disease ecology. He writes:

> It is obvious that as virus host populations (or potential host populations) increase, there is concomitant increase in the probability of major evolutionary changes in virus populations due to increased opportunities for replication, mutation, recombination, and selection. As the world population of humans (and of their domestic animals and plants) increase, the probability for new viral disease outbreaks must inevitably increase as well. AIDS is not the first 'new' virus disease of humans, and it will not be the last.[89]

"From the point of view of a hungry virus," McNeill writes in another piece, "we offer a magnificent feeding ground with all our billions of human bodies, where, in the very recent past, there were only half as many people."[90] (As we shall see later, this same relationship between population density and viral evolution obviously applies to industrial livestock as well.)

How is McNeill's gloomy principle actually woven into the complex fabric of a human-influenced biosphere? In one of the rare studies that has actually attempted to conceptualize the vast web of interconnection between urbanization, the world economy, and the natural environment, an international scientific team recently looked at the implications of the soaring bushmeat trade in West Africa. Their 2004 article in *Science* provides an epistemological model for thinking about influenza emergence in south China and elsewhere.

Explosive city growth in West Africa (where the urban population is expected to reach 60 million by 2025) drives an ever-growing demand for animal protein. Traditionally, West Africans, like many East Asians, have consumed fish as their principal source of protein; fishing, moreover, is a major industry, employing nearly a quarter of the workforce in some countries. But local boats have been unable to compete with the modern, government-subsidized fleets from Europe that now trawl the Gulf of Guinea. These big factory fleets, along with foreign-flag pirate fishers, "illegally extract fish of the highest commercial value, while . . . dumping 70 to 90 percent of their haul as bycatch." As a result fish biomass has fallen by at least half since 1977, and fish has become scarcer and more expensive in local markets. Increasingly bushmeat (the generic name for the flesh of some 400 different species of terrestrial vertebrates) has been substituted for fish—yearly some 400,000 tons of wild game now end up on West African dinner plates. Like the practices that led to declining fish stocks, this level of hunting is unsustainable, and mammal biomass is now decreasing at a rate that fundamentally threatens wildlife diversity.[91]

The authors of this fascinating and troubling study, however, fail to connect a few all-important dots in the causal chain, although undoubtedly they are aware of their importance. One is deforestation, as largely foreign logging companies denude West Africa's remaining coastal rain forests. The bushmeat trade is indissolubly linked to this logging juggernaut and the food needs of its workers, although hunters also poach within official wildlife reserves as well, with the inevitable result being radically increased biological contact between humans and wild animals. The formerly isolated microbiological reservoirs of the rain forests and mountains have been inadvertently integrated into the food economy of the cities—and the result of this "undercurrent of opportunity" has been a series of viral leaps from animals to humans. The most infamous, of course, is HIV/AIDS: researchers believe that HIV-1 arose as a result of humans eating chimpanzees, while HIV-2 (specific to West Africa) has been linked to the consumption of sooty mangabeys. In the fall of 2004 a team headed by Nathan Wolfe of Johns Hopkins raised new fears with the isolation of a novel HIV-like retrovirus (possibly from gorillas) in the bushmeat trade in Cameroon.[92]

There is every reason to believe that the ecological impact of the recent urban-industrial revolution in south China has been just as profound and far-reaching as urban population growth in West Africa. Guangdong—long considered the epicenter of influenza evolution—has become the world's leading export-manufacturing platform, a postmodern Manchester whose toys, running shoes, sports clothing, and cheap electronics are consumed in every corner of the earth. From 1978 until 2002, the province's GDP grew at an astonishing 13.4 percent per year, and the urban population of the Pearl River Delta area increased from 32 percent to 70 percent of the total population. This spectacular regional transformation, crowned by the return of Hong Kong to China in 1997, has been accompanied by a series of socioeconomic developments that are also likely to reinforce Guangdong's primacy as a viral exporter.

Key parameters of influenza emergence include human and animal population densities, intensity of contact between different species, and the prevalence of chronic respiratory or immune disorders. Population densities are very high in the Delta, with about 1,273 persons per square kilometer. A large segment of the population (indeed, the majority in the industrial boomtown of Shenzhen) are rural immigrants or "floaters" in perpetual motion between city factories and thousands of rural villages. Without permanent residency permits, these workers live in overcrowded dormitories or slums and are less likely than the registered population to have access to modern medicine. Meanwhile, the state's share of healthcare spending has fallen sharply (from 34 percent in 1978 to less than 20 percent in 2003) since the advent of a market economy. "[A]bout 50 percent of people who are sick," explains Yanzhong Huang, "do not see a doctor because of the extremely high out-of-pocket payments."[93] And rampant industrialization has increased exposure to all sorts of environmental hazards and toxins. The Delta, for example, has monstrous air pollution: twenty-four times higher than the rest of China. The population accordingly suffers from all the classical respiratory problems (and, probably, cancers) associated with industrial smog and high sulfur dioxide emissions.

Thanks especially to the prevalence of wet markets in the cities, the urbanization of Guangdong has probably intensified rather than decreased microbial traffic between humans and animals. As income has risen with industrial employment, the population is eating more meat and less rice and vegetables. The most dramatic increase has been in the consumption of poultry, which has more than doubled since 1980. Guangdong is one of China's three largest poultry producers and is home to more than *700 million* chickens. An extraordinary concentration of poultry, in other words, coexists with high human densities, large numbers of pigs, and ubiquitous wild birds. Battery chickens, indeed, "are sometimes kept directly above pig pens, depositing their waste right into the pigs' food troughs."[94] Moreover, as the urban footprint has expanded and farm acreage has contracted, a fractal pattern of garden plots next to dormitories and factories has brought urban population and livestock together in more intimate contact. Finally, Guangdong is also a huge market for wild meat. Unlike West Africa, where subsistence demand drives the bushmeat trade, the Chinese predilection for exotic animals stems from ancient homeopathic beliefs; the demand is inexorable, and Laos (via Vietnam) has become a major supplier of live game.[95]

From the beginning of the second wave of H5N1 in the fall of 1997, everyone in Hong Kong was looking nervously over their shoulders at Guangdong and the rest of south China. A newspaper in Beijing reported that there were cases of bird flu in Guangdong but then was forced to retract the story.[96] At the WHO's urging, the CDC sent H5N1 diagnostic kits to researchers in Guangzhou (Canton) and Shenzhen to ensure that everyone doing lab work was using the same protocols. In mid-January, after a brief scuffle over visas, a top-level WHO team was allowed to visit Guangdong for a week. Unlike Hong Kong, with its lively press and political opposition, Guangdong (despite a quarter-million private businesses) was still living under the semantic Maoism of press releases that read, "Thanks to the correct line of the Chinese Communist Party there is no avian flu in Guangdong." Dr. Daniel Lavanchy, at that time the chief influenza expert for WHO, responded in kind with praise for the "high quality of the surveillance activities which had been implemented by the Chinese government." The clear purpose of the mission was to build bridges with provincial and national authorities, not to overturn rocks (or flocks) where H5N1 might be hiding.[97]

The WHO visit bore fruit with the adoption in March of an influenza surveillance plan for south China under the administration of the Chinese National Influenza Center; health workers were asked to be particularly vigilant in reporting and monitoring cases of acute respiratory disease. No human cases of H5N1 were found, but Guangdong and the rest of the south were unexpectedly hit by a severe summer epidemic of normal flu: H3N2. It was a dramatic reminder that influenza can circulate all year round in tropical and semitropical latitudes. In the winter the flu moved north, producing one of the most memorable outbreaks since 1968—in Beijing they called 1998 "the year of the flu."[98] Flu, however, meant H3N2, *not* H5N1. It was almost as if the reigning champion subtype, vintage Hong Kong 1968, had roared back in the face of the brief challenge from the avian usurper.

In a simpler universe, as in some microbiology textbooks, each subtype would patiently await its turn at the helm. But in late winter 1999, the new surveillance system revealed a claim-jumper: Hong Kong scientists were stunned to discover H9N2 in two children in March, with five "officially unconfirmed" cases simultaneously reported from Guangdong. Although none of the cases was life-threatening, the discovery of another hole in the species barrier was unnerving. The new strain was very close to an H9N2 isolated from quail the year before by Guan, Peiris, and Shortridge. But it was not the only H9 in town. Surveillance of pigs in a Hong Kong slaughterhouse found animals with the quail strain as well as some with a distinctive H9N2 derived from ducks. Genetic analysis then implicated the H9 quail strain in the viral *ménage à trois* that had generated the 1997 killer. The internal proteins in H5N1 were virtually identical with those from H9N2.[99]

With this double recognition that H9N2 was a precursor of H5N1 reassortment, as well as a human invader in its own right, the story was getting surprisingly messy. Nonlinear complexity now governed the plot. As some theorists had already recognized, the "interactive dynamics" between multiple, coevolving subtypes might "introduce complexities and substantial mathematical challenges" that would make modeling or predicting viral evolution extraordinarily difficult, if not impossible.[100] To gain a better understanding of what was actually happening, the University of Hong Kong research team headed by Guan, Peiris, and Shortridge decided to explore the viral underworld of Guangdong in unprecedented detail. They wanted to find out how many subtypes and strains were circulating in the avian population and, most importantly, how they were interacting with one another. For a year, starting in July 2000, researchers carefully isolated viruses from ducks in the live-poultry markets of the Guangdong city of Shantou. The results of their study, published in the summer of 2003, fundamentally revised the standard picture of influenza evolution.

First of all, they discovered extraordinary and unexpected genetic diversity: almost 500 distinct strains of influenza, including fifty-three different iterations of the H9 subtype. "The diversity of genotypes, gene constellations, and host receptor specificities," they warned, "will provide these viruses and their progeny with options of hosts." Second, they established that reassortment was a more common event than previously imagined. Gene segments were vigorously being traded throughout the diverse network of influenzas. Previously, "influenza gene flow was usually considered to occur from aquatic birds to other animals." Now they found ample evidence that viruses were evolving from ducks to poultry and back again: "i.e., there is a two-way transmission between terrestrial and aquatic." "The species barriers between the birds have become much more permeable than previously anticipated. Increasing the heterogeneity of influenza viruses in these hosts results in an enlarged and dynamic influenza gene pool in continuous flux rather than one that is limited to aquatic birds and therefore in evolutionary stasis."[101] Or, as American virologist Richard Webby pithily put it, "we have a bucket of evolution going on."[102]

The bottom-line of the Shantou report was that several subtypes of influenza were traveling on the path toward pandemic potential. The industrialization of south China, perhaps, had altered crucial parameters in an already very complex ecological system, exponentially expanding the surface area of contact between avian and nonavian influenzas. As the rate of interspecies transmission of influenza accelerated, so too did the evolution of protopandemic strains. The Hong Kong research team had discovered, in other words, that contemporary influenza, like a postmodern novel, has no single narrative, but rather disparate storylines racing one another to dictate a bloody conclusion. "The H5N1 virus was in the process of adapting from aquatic to land-based poultry from the duck via the partially aquatic goose to the chicken," while the H9N2 (and probably H6N1) were "adapting through a mechanism that took them to the quail and probably other minor land-based poultry such as the pheasant." Alternately, "aquatic migratory or domestic birds could introduce a 'genetically adaptable' virus directly into land-based poultry. The intensification of the poultry industry through large-scale commercial operations in East Asia (and elsewhere) could facilitate this."[103]

Each of the aspirant subtypes had different assets. If H5N1 was an assassin of unparalleled lethality, the fact that H9N1 strains—according to the Hong Kong team—were "not highly pathogenic for poultry . . . makes them more, rather than less, likely to be of pandemic relevance." A milder chicken virus was more likely to survive detection and extermination and thus have time to continue to reassort until it found the optimal gene constellation for rapid infection of human populations.[104] In 2003 the Hong Kong researchers would find further evidence to corroborate the pandemic potential of H9N2 in a study of viruses in the live-poultry markets of their own city.[105]

Meanwhile, H5N1 was again laying siege to Hong Kong. Between February and March 2001, the surveillance network found several strains of the virus among market chickens, quail, pheasants, and pigeons. A few months later, South Korean authorities isolated H5N1 in imported Chinese duck meat. Laboratory testing subsequently revealed that these H5N1 genotypes were a separate reassortment from the 1997 strain and had most likely originated sometime in late 2000 from goose viruses that had "crossed to ducks and re-assorted with other unknown influenza viruses of aquatic origin." Researchers were

horrified to discover that the new H5N1 was even more pathogenic than the old: when mice were infected with the 2001
strains, the virus spread to the brain and killed the animals. In
May chickens started dying again in the city's markets, and
once more the city government mandated a slaughter of local
poultry before the new strains infected humans or reassorted
with H9N2.[106]

With so much heavy genetic traffic between feral avian reservoirs, domestic poultry, and mammals, researchers were becoming
pessimistic about the likelihood of successfully containing further
outbreaks by local culling of birds. When H5N1 returned again
in February 2002, top virologist Yi Guan of the University of
Hong Kong told *China Daily* that truly drastic action was now
necessary—live poultry had to go. Guan said, "I believe that we
have to get rid of the farms, and the poultry markets, and the import of fresh chickens." The poultry industry—seemingly obliv-
ious to the nature of the pandemic threat—screamed that the
scientists had gone berserk. "Avian influenza is just like any human flu—you just cannot get rid of it. However, it does not make
sense to get rid of the poultry industry to get rid of the bird flu.
That would be an ignorant act."[107] The authorities seemingly
agreed, and they restricted their response to ordering the destruction of another 900,000 chickens.

In December, textbook theory was again confounded as
H5N1 began to decimate its natural hosts. Ducks, as well as geese,
flamingos, swans, egrets, and herons, started dying in two popular
Hong Kong parks; mallards—presumed immune to the pathogenic effects of influenza—developed catastrophic neurological
disorders. The dead ducks were incontrovertible proof that a two-
way flow of H5N1 mutants now existed between aquatic and

terrestrial birds. Researchers who studied the outbreak were troubled by the theoretical implications:

> A pathogenic H5N1 outbreak among waterfowl and wild birds is therefore novel and has serious implications. . . . Previous phylogenetic studies had shown low evolutionary rates of avian influenza viruses in waterfowl. Therefore, it was generally accepted that influenza viruses were in evolutionary stasis in wild aquatic birds, with no evidence of clear evolution over the past 60 years. The data presented in this paper raise the possibility that this balance may be changing in ducks or that it has been disrupted by the introduction of novel viruses to ducks from some other avian source.[108]

Scientists worried that antigenic drift had been accelerated by the illegal use of unregistered poultry vaccines in Guangdong. Other researchers speculated that lethal strains of H5N1 might spread through the wild duck population and follow the annual migration back to Siberian or even Alaskan lakes.[109] (In 2004, the United Nations' Food and Agriculture Organization [FAO] learned that Russian researchers in Novosibirsk had indeed found H5N1—95 percent similar to the Hong Kong strain—the previous year in a wild mallard duck on Lake Chany in western Siberia.)[110] In any event, as Shortridge, Peiris, and Guan glumly pointed out in an article, it was now evident that the H5N1 infection in birds had become "non-eradicable."[111] Meanwhile, Hong Kong closed its parks and slaughtered its beloved wild birds.

Two months later, at the beginning of February 2003, a seven-year-old girl died of an acute respiratory disease while visiting a Fujian province in the company of her mother, sister, and brother. She was buried before the exact cause of death could be ascertained. Her father, who rushed from Hong Kong to his dying daughter's bedside, was also stricken and died in mid-February, nine days after his return to Hong Kong; his eight-year-old son developed critical symptoms of respiratory distress but ultimately recovered.[112] Both father and son were confirmed to have been infected with the same strain of H5N1 that was killing ducks in the parks. Genetic sequencing revealed that it was a remote cousin to the original 1997 strain. The hemagglutinin was derived from the same lineage, but the internal proteins and neuraminidase had evolved elsewhere. Some researchers surmised that the influenza had been contracted in Fujian—the family's relatives kept chickens—and were skeptical of China's claim that it had not experienced any large-scale outbreaks of avian influenza among ducks or poultry.[113] In any event, experts were troubled by further evidence of increasing virulence in the rapidly evolving H5N1 family. WHO went to pandemic alert status, and public-health officials again buckled their seatbelts.

6

Pandemic Surprise

Humankind has had a lucky escape.[114]

Robin Weiss and Angela McLean

Shortly before the isolation of the new avian-to-human H5N1 in Hong Kong in 2003, the WHO office in Beijing received an email warning that a "strange contagious disease" had killed more than one hundred people in Guangdong in a single week. Medical workers and foodhandlers were said to be especially affected. In the provincial capital of Guangzhou (Canton), panicked residents were buying up surgical masks and antibiotics as well as white vinegar, a traditional folk treatment for respiratory illness. Over the next few days, Chinese public-health officials grudgingly acknowledged that five people had died from "atypical pneumonia"; the outbreak had started in Foshan the previous November, had infected about 300 people, but was now "under control." The Chinese were admitting, in effect, that they had concealed the epidemic from the WHO, but were now urging the world "not to worry"—they emphasized that the victims had all tested negative for influenza. But provincial and national authorities gave conflicting accounts of the likely pathogen: Guangdong blamed the bacterium *Mycoplasma pneumoniae,* while Beijing insisted that it was actually *Chlamydia.* To further erode credibility, "a spokesman for the Guangdong health department told reporters that all further information would be disseminated by the party propaganda unit."[115] Although these prohibitions did not stop the Internet from gushing rumors, authorities also threatened that "any physician or journalist who reported on the disease would risk being persecuted for leaking state secrets."[116]

Veteran influenza researchers were highly skeptical of the official Chinese account. With avian influenza again killing birds in Hong Kong, it was logical to suspect that the mysterious pneumonia was, in fact, the beginning of the long-dreaded pandemic. The reports from Guangdong, moreover, were soon followed by the identification of the two, possibly three, human H5N1 cases: could this be just a coincidence? Circumstantial evidence supported the worst-case scenario. It also followed that if the disease were in Hong Kong, south China's portal to the world, the virus might escape on the first available plane.

As investigators later reconstructed the itinerary, this is exactly what happened in the third week of February. A doctor from Guangzhou who had been attending victims of the pneumonia, arrived in Hong Kong on 21 February for a family wedding. Already ill, he checked into a room on the ninth floor of the Metropole Hotel, where by some unidentified mechanism, he managed to transmit his virus to sixteen other guests on the same floor—in the parlance of epidemiology, the doctor was a "superspreader." As the infected hotel guests, including airline crew members, traveled onward to other destinations, they quickly transformed the Guangdong outbreak into an embryonic global pandemic. The CDC would later construct a flowchart of cases that originated from the Metropole Hotel: 195 in

Hong Kong, 71 in Singapore, 58 in Vietnam, 29 in Canada, and 1 each in Ireland and the United States. As WHO Global Outbreak Alert and Response scientists later marveled, "A global outbreak was thus seeded from a single person on a single day on a single floor of a Hong Kong hotel."[117]

The first Metropole case to attract WHO attention was a Chinese-American businessman who became desperately ill in Hanoi. Local hospital staff, petrified by the possibility that it was a case of avian flu, asked the local WHO representative, Dr. Carlo Urbani, to oversee the patient. The Italian doctor alerted the WHO Regional Office for the Western Pacific on 28 February that the mystery disease was now a traveler, and there were soon outbreaks in several other countries. On 1 March, with several patients already hospitalized in Hong Kong, a female flight attendant (the first of several Metropole victims) was admitted to a Singapore hospital with acute respiratory distress. A few days later, an elderly Canadian who had stayed in the Metropole died in Toronto, and five members of her family were soon hospitalized. Meanwhile, in a pattern that confirmed rumors from Guangdong, hospital workers who had been exposed to the Metropole patients in Hong Kong and Hanoi developed symptoms; the French Hospital in Hanoi was forced to close. Next, the Chinese-American businessman died, followed by the son of the elderly Toronto woman. By mid-March, scores of medical personnel in Hanoi and Hong Kong were in intensive care, and Ontario officials had to seal off Scarborough Grace Hospital. Dr. Urbani developed the disease and was evacuated from Hanoi to a hospital in Thailand, where he died on 29 March. By this time, some frightened hospital staff in China, Canada, and Vietnam refused to treat patients diagnosed with the enigmatic, deadly illness.

Was it avian influenza? The pathogen was still unidentified on 15 March when the WHO labeled the disease after its symptoms: Severe Acute Respiratory Syndrome or SARS. On that same day, a young Singaporean physician, returning from a medical conference in New York, was hospitalized during a stopover in Frankfurt along with his pregnant wife and mother-in-law. The doctor had treated the stewardess in Singapore: another superspreader, she would ultimately be the source of almost one hundred other cases. Although WHO finally issued a warning to the airline industry, it came too late to prevent other infected passengers from subsequently carrying SARS to Beijing and Taiwan. At the end of March, both Hong Kong and Toronto authorities were pressed to take more drastic action. Hong Kong officials closed schools and put more than 1,080 residents under quarantine, while in Toronto, another hospital was closed off and thousands of hospital workers and others in contact with SARS cases were asked to quarantine themselves at home.

In Hong Kong the epidemic assumed nightmarish proportions in the Amoy Gardens housing complex in Kowloon. Tower Block E was thirty-three stories high with eight apartments on each floor; the virus was first brought to the building in mid-March by a resident's brother, who had recently undergone dialysis at the SARS-infected Prince of Wales Hospital. He was suffering badly from diarrhea and used his brother's toilet. Within a few days, an extraordinary 321 residents of Block E and adjoining buildings developed SARS. The mode of transmission remains a mystery. Although some experts insist that the contagion had to be airborne (perhaps as residents shared elevators), Department of Health officials concluded that SARS was disseminated, at least in part, through faulty plumbing that brought residents "into contact with small droplets containing viruses from the contaminated sewage." The Amoy Gardens incident was particularly troubling because it demonstrated that in conditions of extreme urban density—such as those found in high-rise housing, hospitals, and slums—viral transmission might be potently amplified by faulty ventilation and sewage systems, or, worse, by those systems' absence.[118]

Meanwhile, SARS had become a test of China's international credibility, with Health Minister Zhang Wenkang continuing to antagonize the world public-health community with his perfunctory and reliably inaccurate reports on the epidemic. Since early February, WHO experts had urgently wanted to visit Guangdong to investigate conditions there, but the Health Ministry obstructed the mission until the beginning of April—by then, SARS has set Beijing ablaze as well. China's "official secrets" law had prevented Guangdong officials from briefing other local health authorities about the disease, so when the first cases appeared in Beijing in early March, local doctors were clueless. When the WHO team flew to Beijing, they were initially blocked from inspecting the military hospitals where most of the victims were being treated. Although officials continued to assert that the epidemic was contained, on 16 April WHO took the unprecedented step of chastising the Chinese government for "inadequate reporting" of SARS cases.[119]

Chinese leaders were deeply worried about the impact of the epidemic upon trade and economic growth. SARS, says Yanzhong Huang in a fascinating account, "caused the most severe socio-political crisis for the Chinese leadership since the 1989 Tiananmen crackdown." China's still-powerful former president, Jiang Zemin, reputedly urged strict censorship, while his successor, Hu Jintao, favored disclosure and collaboration with the WHO. Old-guard Beijing officials tried to conceal the full extent of the new epidemic not only from the outside world but even from high-ranking officials in the Zemin faction. When the WHO, for the first time in its history, advised visitors to stay away from Hong Kong and Guangdong, the Health Minister responded that SARS had been contained and that south China was completely safe for visitors. A courageous whistle-blower, a retired military surgeon named Jiang Yanyong who had treated many victims of the Tiananmen Square massacre, circulated an email that accused the minister of bald-faced lying.* *Time* magazine covered the story and, according to Huang, "triggered a political earthquake in Beijing."[120]

President Hu Jintao and his supporters now took firm command of the situation: bureaucratic duplicity and inaction were replaced by an almost Maoist display of party-state willpower. The equivalent of 1 billion dollars in state aid (a fraction of the economic damage already caused to China and Hong Kong) was made available to upgrade local hospitals and public-health services. Health Minister Zhang Wenkang and Beijing Mayor Meng Xuenong—both Zemin loyalists—were purged, and other officials were bluntly told that their survival depended upon extirpating SARS. "Driven by political zeal, they sealed off villages, apartment complexes, and university campuses, quarantined tens of thousands of people, and set up checkpoints to take temperatures. . . . In Guangdong, 80 million people were mobilized to clean houses and streets. In the

---

* The ever doughty Jiang was subsequently arrested in June 2004 after circulating a letter asking the government to apologise for the Tiananmen massacre.

countryside, virtually every village was on SARS alert, with roadside booths installed to examine all those who entered or left." To the surprise of many, these draconian quarantines— "momentous measures" says Yanzhong Huang—seemed to work. The spread of the SARS epidemic inside China was arrested, and in late June the WHO canceled its warnings about travel to Hong Kong and Beijing.[121]

While the drama inside China was unfolding, a WHO-organized virtual consortium of laboratories was working night and day to discover the cause of SARS. Within a month, this unprecedented research effort, spearheaded by Malik Peiris and his colleagues in Hong Kong and Shenzhen, had isolated a coronavirus. Although scientists were greatly relieved that it was not "the Big One" (an influenza pandemic) after all, they were flabbergasted that a member of a viral family normally associated with mild colds and diarrhea had become an international serial killer. And as researchers sequenced the genome of the SARS virus, they found little link to any of the known human-adapted members of the family. The SARS virus was genetically *sui generis*.

There was much speculation about an exotic animal source. Once again, the crack Hong Kong team led by Guan, Peiris, and Shortridge returned to the wet markets, this time in Shenzhen, the boomtown neighbor of Hong Kong. Among caged animals in the retail wildlife market, they soon found the SARS virus in a group of masked palm civets and a raccoon dog; a Chinese ferret badger also showed evidence of SARS' antibodies.[122] All three small carnivores are considered luxury or health items in the diet of Guangdong urban dwellers. (Ironically, civets are eaten because of a homeopathic belief that they provide immunity to influenza.)

They are also lucrative commodities in the booming south China bushmeat trade that includes imports from Laos and Vietnam. SARS, then, like HIV, was a deadly by-product of a largely illegal international wildlife trade, intimately connected with logging and deforestation, which mortally threatens human health as well as regional biodiversity.[123]

The WHO officially declared the SARS outbreaks contained on 5 July. (A small-scale outbreak at the end of 2003, quickly controlled by Chinese authorities, reminded the world that SARS will be a recurrent danger until the prototype vaccine, now being field-tested, becomes widely available.) The first pandemic of the twenty-first century had generated approximately 8,500 cases in 26 countries; nearly 11 percent of SARS patients (916) died worldwide, although mortality in some localities was closer to 20 percent. Like influenza, SARS had a very strong preference for the elderly, whose death rate was over 50 percent. Young adults, in contrast, had only a 7 percent chance of dying, while SARS was seldom life-threatening to children.[124]

The management of the epidemic in Hong Kong and Toronto—each with an identical death rate of 17 percent—was the subject of investigation by expert panels in both cities. A summary of their respective findings was published in 2004 by the *Journal of the American Medical Association* (*JAMA*). As the panel chairs emphasize: "Both areas were hampered by underinvestment in public-health infrastructure, diminution of public-health leadership, and weak links between health care and public health." In both cities, moreover, the health systems were overwhelmed by the epidemic. No one had expected a disease that targeted hospitals or took such a heavy toll on primary health-care personnel:

22 percent of SARS cases in Hong Kong, 43 percent in Toronto. Early in the Guangdong outbreak, some 90 percent of cases were among health-care workers. The Ontario government had to import, more or less clandestinely, several hundred U.S. doctors to make up the shortfall caused by ill or frightened physicians. In Hong Kong the hospital system almost broke down because of the lack of infection control in emergency rooms and the shortage of isolation units (single, negative-pressure rooms). In any event, *JAMA* reported, "neither jurisdiction had enough infection control practitioners and infectious disease specialists." The distressing spread of SARS among medical personnel, however, was not due to the virus's super-infectivity, but, rather, to surprisingly widespread failure of hospital staff to adhere to proper protective clothing and standard hygiene (such as simple hand-washing). In both cities, lines of authority were blurred or contradictory, and general practitioners were often left totally in the dark about diagnostic and therapeutic procedures. In the end, the nineteenth century, not the twenty-first, defeated SARS: "containment of SARS relied heavily on application of public health and clinical infection-control measures rooted in nineteenth-century science."[125]

The laboratory manipulation of SARS also revealed dangerous flaws in the biosecurity of many research institutes and universities working with respiratory viruses. In separate incidents in Singapore and Taiwan, researchers managed to infect themselves with SARS. Robert Webster cited these cases in a January 2004 *Lancet* article in which he warned that an influenza pandemic might start with the escape of a dangerous fossil virus such as H2N2, the 1957 pandemic strain against which no one born since 1968 has any immunity. He reminded readers that the sudden reappearance of H1N1 in 1977, after a twenty-year hiatus, was probably the result of a lab accident in Russia or China.[126]

The SARS outbreak has also been studied as a real-life test of the preparedness of world organizations, national governments, and local health systems to respond to an influenza pandemic. "The quick and effective response of the WHO to SARS," reported British experts to the Royal Society, "did much to restore faith among the many critics of the effectiveness of international agencies with large bureaucracies and limited resources for action." But they warned that the successful containment of the SARS pandemic had sowed the illusion that the "system works," when, in their view, the system was simply "very lucky." The "simple public health measures that worked well for SARS" are "unlikely to be effective" in the case of an "antigenically novel influenza virus, of both high pathogenicity and transmissibility." "Sentiments of the type 'we have been successful once—we will be again' may be far from the truth."[127]

What are the key differences between SARS and influenza? Although SARS produces similar symptoms, it is not nearly as "subtle" as influenza.[128] As Peiris and Guan emphasize, "SARS manifested several features that made it more amenable to control through public health measures than some other potential emerging infectious disease threats."[129] In the first place, SARS needs about five days to incubate and does not usually become contagious until well after the onset of fever and dry coughing; infectiousness takes about ten days to peak, and research has found few asymptomatic infections without sickness. The old-fashioned tactics of isolation and quarantine, if ruthlessly implemented, can work effectively against such a slow-developing virus whose symptoms consistently signal infectiousness.

Influenza is an altogether different story. It is fast and deceptive, and infectiousness and sickness do not coincide; an infected person massively sheds virus and becomes highly contagious a day or more before the actual onset of symptoms. (HIV, with its long, silent incubation period is, of course, even more insidious because the infected person can be contagious for years without manifesting any symptoms or sickness.) Moreover, influenza epidemics include large numbers of asymptomatic infections: spreaders without symptoms. Influenza, as a result, is more transmissible. In addition, technically it has a higher "R" or "basic reproduction number" (defined as the "average number of secondary cases generated by one primary case in a susceptible population") than does SARS, or for that matter, HIV. A typical flu has an R of 5 to 25 while SARS is only 2 to 3 (not counting the still poorly understood phenomenon of so-called superspreaders). To stop an epidemic of SARS, public-health officials need only block viral transmission, either by isolation or quarantine, in about half the cases. Control of pandemic flu, on the other hand, requires an almost 100 percent containment of infection.[130] Traditional isolation measures, accordingly, may not be much more effective tomorrow than they were in 1918.

Finally, the 2002–3 SARS pandemic had a fortuitous geography. China and Singapore were both authoritarian states with the capacity to impose effective, militarized quarantines. (In Singapore this took the Orwellian form of temperature-detecting sensors in the airport and home video-surveillance of hundreds of quarantined individuals.) Guangdong, moreover, by Chinese standards is a rich region with a much more modern health-care infrastructure than poorer inland provinces. Although SARS exposed the Achilles heel of neglect and underinvestment in their public-health systems, Toronto and Hong Kong are likewise affluent cities with superb laboratory medicine.

SARS in Bangladesh, Afghanistan, or Zaire would have been a different pandemic. This is exactly the "What if?" that haunted the Royal Society's postmortem on the SARS pandemic: "[S]uppose the virus had flown from Hong Kong to Durban instead of Toronto. It is a city of similar size but without a similar health infrastructure, and with a significant proportion of its inhabitants immune-compromised owing to HIV-1 infection. Then Africa could have become endemic for SARS by now."[131] An influenza pandemic, to be sure, would not neglect the poor countries of the world.

7

The Triangle of Doom

We need to look in our own backyard for where the next pandemic may appear.[132]

Christopher Olsen

The SARS pandemic ratified Guangdong's exceptional importance as a disease epicenter. But does Guangdong have a unique franchise? Some influenza experts believe that all pandemics originate in the mixed swine-and-poultry agriculture of south China, a near-dogma that makes them resist compelling evidence that the 1918 reassortant first emerged in Kansas.[133] Other researchers, however, argue that the environmental preconditions for the rapid interspecies evolution of influenza are now found elsewhere, and they point specifically to the ecological impacts of the export-led industrialization of poultry and pork production since the 1980s.

This so-called Livestock Revolution has been primarily driven by Third World urbanization and the rising demand in developing countries—above all, China—for poultry, pork, and dairy products. Although Third World urban dwellers are obviously poorer than their OECD counterparts, a much larger percentage of income growth is expended on animal protein, and this is the demand engine that currently drives huge

81

increases in chicken and swine populations. According to Australian researchers, "The [global] share of meat and milk consumed in developing countries rose from 37 to 53 percent and from 34 to 44 percent, respectively, from 1983 to 1997. . . . By contrast, both per capita and aggregate milk and meat consumption stagnated in the developed world, where saturation levels of consumption have been reached and population growth is small." From the standpoint of influenza ecology, moreover, it is striking that pork and poultry constitute 76 percent of the developing world's increased meat consumption, and poultry has accounted for almost all of the small net

Table 7.1.
The Livestock Revolution[134]

(million metric tons)

	1983	1997	2020
DEVELOPED WORLD			
Total meat	88	99	117
Pork	34	36	39
Poultry	19	28	39
THIRD WORLD			
Total meat	50	112	217
Pork	20	46	81
Poultry	10	29	70
CHINA			
Total meat	16	53	107

increase in rich countries' food consumption.[135] The viral "food supply"—poultry, swine, and humans—has been dramatically enlarged.

Like the Green Revolution before it, the Livestock Revolution has favored corporate producers rather than peasants and family farmers. As a recent UN report emphasizes, "large-scale, industrial production accounts already for roughly 80 percent of the total production increase in livestock products in Asia since 1990. In the future, most production, especially of pigs and poultry, is expected not to come from traditional production systems that have characterized the region for centuries, but from industrial, large-scale production."[136]

The world icon of industrialized poultry and livestock production is giant Tyson Foods, which, like Wal-Mart, grew up in hardscrabble Arkansas. Tyson, which kills 2.2 billion chickens annually, has become globally synonymous with scaled-up, vertically coordinated production; exploitation of contract growers; visceral antiunionism; rampant industrial injury; downstream environmental dumping; and political corruption. The global dominance of behemoths like Tyson has forced local farmers to either integrate with large-scale chicken- and pork-processing firms or perish. "These firms," write Donald Stull and Michael Broadway, "owned not only the broilers they supplied to contract growers, but the eggs that hatched the birds, the feed that went into them, and the plants that processed and then sold them to grocery stores."[137] Whether in the Ozarks, Holland, or Thailand, entire farming districts have been converted to the warehousing of poultry, with farmers serving as little more than chicken custodians. At the same time, livestock has been disintegrated from agriculture; thus creating a new geography where grain and feed production is spatially separate from the raising of chickens and pigs.[138]

The result has been extraordinary population concentrations of poultry. A crucial requirement of the modern chicken industry, for example, is "production density," the compact location of broiler farms around a large processing plant.[139] As a result, there are now regions in North America, Brazil, western Europe, and South Asia with chicken populations in the hundreds of millions—in western Arkansas and northern Georgia, for example, more than 1 billion chickens are slaughtered annually. Similarly, the raising of swine is increasingly centralized in huge operations, often adjacent to poultry farms and migratory bird habitats. The superurbanization of the human population, in other words, has been paralleled by an equally dense urbanization of its meat supply. (One swine megafarm in Milford Valley, Utah, reputedly produces more sewage than the city of Los Angeles.) Might not one of these artificial Guangdongs be a pandemic crucible as well? Could production density become a synonym for viral density?

The answer to these questions was revealed in March of 2003. While scientists were desperately trying to figure out the identity of an atypical pneumonia in China, chickens were dying on a farm in the Gelder Valley (Gelderland) of Holland. The Netherlands is the world's leading exporter of eggs and live chickens, as well as a major producer of turkeys and geese; the hundreds of chicken farms in the Gelderland are at the center of the highly rationalized, $2 billion-per-year Dutch poultry industry. Many of the farms also keep pet flocks of ducks and swans.[140] With its intimate juxtaposition of wetlands, wild birds, poultry, and high urban density, as well as its hub-like role in the

European Union's global commerce, the Netherlands recapitulates many of the distinctive features of the Pearl River Delta; the March epidemic, in fact, was later traced back to a farm whose free-range chickens were in contact with wild waterfowl in an adjacent canal.

Although vigilant Dutch agricultural authorities quickly quarantined the movement of chickens and temporarily halted poultry exports, the Highly Pathogenic Avian Influenza (HPAI) swept like wildfire through the Gelderland. The virus was identified as an H7N7 strain more or less identical to a strain isolated in mallards several years earlier.[141] By April, turkeys were dying in North Brabant, and the first HPAI cases were reported in Meeuwen-Gruitrode in neighboring Belgium. Even more disturbingly, evidence of the infection was discovered in pigs on several farms in the Gelderland, increasing the dangerous likelihood of H7N7's reassortment with swine and human influenzas. (The pigs were promptly slaughtered.) As European Union agricultural experts fretted over the potential for a pan-European epidemic, the Dutch government came under immense domestic and foreign pressure to act more aggressively. The Hague decided to exterminate all the poultry in the Gelderland and other infected areas and to dispose of thousands of tons of virus-laden chicken manure. As thousands of unhappy farmers clamored in protest, crews of poultry workers, aided by the Dutch army, began the epic slaughter of more than 30 million chickens, almost one-third of Holland's entire poultry population.[142]

Although HPAI was an enormous threat to the poultry industry, there was little apprehension of any public-health danger. A few years earlier, there had been a serious H7N7 outbreak among chickens in Italy, but serological analysis found no evidence of any transmission to humans. Moreover, all the personnel involved in the Dutch cull wore protective clothing, including goggles and mouth-and-nose masks. Even when a veterinarian who been involved in the early identification of the outbreak developed acute conjunctivitis, experts expressed surprise but not alarm: in 1996, an English duck owner had developed mild conjunctivitis after contact with a sick bird and there was an extraordinary case where an avian H7 had been transmitted to a human from a sick seal, but did not cause serious illness; H7N7 was also known to be endemic in horses. The virus's modest talent for crossing species barriers had never been accompanied by corresponding virulence—on rare occasions the virus apparently could inflame cells around the eye but it had shown no ability to replicate in the human respiratory tract or other tissues.[143]

This benign view of H7N7, however, was quickly challenged by a chorus of complaints from poultry workers with conjunctivitis, and in a few cases, reports of classical flu symptoms. Because some immigrant workers, now unemployed after the cull, had already returned to their native countries, there was concern that they might seed new outbreaks. The prestigious Dutch National Institute of Public Health and the Environment quickly dispatched an expert investigation team, under the leadership of Dr. Marion Koopmans, to the Gelderland. A medical command center was established, and from 8 March nurses visited every household that might have had contact with infected birds. Since the ordinary flu season was in progress, vaccinations were made obligatory for poultry workers and their families, although this policy was implemented too late to prevent several worrisome cases of co-infection by H7N7 and normal H3N1. Meanwhile, the outbreak team was stunned by the scale of infection they discovered: 553 people out of an exposed population of approximately 4,500 reported conjunctivitis or other symptoms; subsequent serological studies demonstrated that, in fact, as many as 2,000 of the exposed group had been infected but not always sickened. Surgical masks and goggles, for whatever reason, had afforded the poultry cullers little or no protection against the virus.[144]

Moreover, relatives and housemates of poultry workers, who had no direct contact with infected birds, also developed conjunctivitis. Public-health officials were convinced that the virus had acquired a limited but real ability to spread via person-to-person contact, although the exact mode of transmission was unclear. The outbreak team also found evidence that H7N7 was accumulating dangerous mutations as it passed through the human population. The event's most frightening moment was the death of a fifty-seven-year-old veterinarian on 19 April; soon after exposure to sick chickens, he had developed viral pneumonia (and later ARDS) instead of relatively benign conjunctivitis. Previously in good health, he was not immune-compromised, nor did he have any underlying disease. Alarmingly, his catastrophic decline matched the gruesome clinical descriptions of the 1997 deaths in Hong Kong, or for that matter, the acute cases in 1918.[145]

An urgent analysis of viral samples removed from the vet's lungs revealed that the strain that killed him was not an avian–human reassortant, as some had feared, but a variant of the original H7N7 virus which had undergone twelve amino acid substitutions; some mutations affected its hemagglutinin, while others modified the PB2 protein, part of the polymerase complex that helped replicate the virus. While HA has always been influenza's celebrity protein because of its crucial role in determining host range, and possibly, virulence, the Dutch researchers, like colleagues elsewhere, were coming around to the idea that mutations in internal proteins—such as PB2 or the nonstructural protein NS2—might be important co-factors in the severity of infection. They knew that previous research had shown that a mutation in PB2 had increased the virulence of H5N1 in mice—perhaps H7N7 reacted the same way. In any event, the Dutch outbreak, with its deadly index case, now had the WHO's attention, even if the world press was diverted by the ongoing battle against SARS.[146]

After H7N7's brief forays into Belgium and Germany, the outbreak was officially contained in August. Dutch experts regarded it as another harrowingly close call with a potentially deadly pandemic:

> Although we launched a large and costly outbreak investigation (using a combination of pandemic and bioterrorism preparedness protocols), and despite decisions being made very quickly, a sobering conclusion is that by the time full prophylactic measures were reinforced . . . more than 1000 people from all over the Netherlands and from abroad had been exposed. Therefore if a variant with more effective spreading capabilities had arisen, containment would have been very difficult.[147]

Like the earlier H9 outbreak, the Gelderland epidemic demonstrated that multiple subtypes (including H9, H7, and possibly

H4 and H6, as well as reborn H2) were racing H5 to the pandemic finish line. The rapidity and scale of the Dutch outbreak also proved that south China no longer had a monopoly on deadly influenza: there were now multiple epicenters.

The H7N7 crisis also provided an additional reason for public-health officials and human influenza researchers to talk to their expert animal-virus counterparts. In the past, human and veterinary medicines had been parallel sciences that only occasionally intersected during rare interspecies disease events, but now the two viral universes, animal and human, seem to be locked together in a frenetic evolutionary embrace that makes the old dualism seem obsolete. Let me suggest an analogy: during the Second World War, the Allies and Nazis fought a secret high-stakes war over remote weather stations in Greenland, because knowledge of weather-front conditions in East Greenland anticipated Western Europe's weather by several days; such intelligence was of incalculable value in planning strategic surprises such as D-Day or the Battle of the Bulge. Likewise, the March 2003 Dutch epidemic proved how crucial veterinary surveillance has become for anticipating human outbreaks. To avoid a catastrophic pandemic surprise, it is urgent to know what is happening on farms months, even years, ahead of any human transmission.

Several specific developments in the wake of the global Livestock Revolution have especially put scientists' nerves on edge. One is the sudden viral chaos on pig farms since 1997. For the previous sixty or seventy years, swine influenza—a lineage derived from the H1N1 of 1918—exhibited extraordinary genetic stability. Although individual pigs occasionally became mixing vessels for avian strains (as many believed happened in 1957 and again in 1968), the H1N1 dynasty was otherwise as unremitting as the Habsburgs. Then in 1997, the hogs on one of North Carolina's megafarms caught H3N2, a human flu; this subtype soon reassorted with avian and classic swine viruses, and "by late 1999, the novel viruses could be found wherever there were pigs in North America and so were presumably spread by cross-country transport." The emergent menagerie includes an H1N2 that is the offspring of human and swine subtypes, as well as an H1N1 that preserves the classical outer proteins but whose internal proteins are human and avian. All novel subtypes are dangerous, but an H4N6 virus, a wholly avian strain that passed to Canadian hogs from ducks, is perhaps the most sinister, because it has "already acquired genetic mutations that give it the potential to bind to human cell receptors." "Such an event," warns one research team, "could be catastrophic, as humans have no immunity to H4 viruses."[148]

The new swine flu pandemic threat apparently has arisen directly from the increasing scale of hog production; researchers told *Science* that swine influenza's sudden burst of mutational energy has probably been stimulated by parallel changes in herd size, interstate transport of hogs, and vaccination practice. Since 1993, U.S. pork production has been restructured around the Tyson, or "poultry model," of very large, industrialized units. In a single decade, from 1993 to 2003, the percentage of hogs raised on factory farms with more than 5,000 animals increased from 18 percent to 53 percent. Such large herds maximize the opportunities for new viruses to replicate and develop epidemic momentum. "With a group of 5000 animals," an agricultural statistician explained to *Science*, "if a novel virus shows up, it will have more opportunity to replicate and potentially spread than in a group of 100 pigs on a small farm."[149]

Increased shipping of hogs over distance simultaneously expands the radius of potential infection. Meanwhile, "in less than a decade, vaccination has become the norm for breeding sows, which in turn pass their maternal antibodies on to their progeny . . . but the vaccine is not protecting against all new strains." What seems to be happening, instead, is that influenza vaccinations—like the notorious antibiotics given to steers—are probably selecting for resistant new viral types. In the absence of any official surveillance system for swine flu, a dangerous reassortant could emerge with little warning.[150]

Another "in our own backyard" trend that raises anxiety is the prevalence of so-called Low Pathogenic Avian Influenza (LPAI); LPAI infections, according to the *Terrestrial Animal Health Code* published by the Office International des Epizooties (OIE), are endemic in wild birds, causing mild symptoms and low mortality in poultry. In the United States, the Department of Agriculture responds to all HPAI outbreaks, but control of LPAI is left to individual states whose agricultural agencies are often captives of local agribusiness. In an era of crumbling species barriers and increasing pandemic risk, such special-interest federalism poses unacceptable public-health risks: consider the secret LPAI epidemic in California in 2000–4.

In 2000 an H6N2 influenza began circulating in Southern California poultry. The virus intrigued the scientists who sequenced its genome, because its proteins appeared to derive from both North American and Eurasian lineages of waterfowl: this was considered to be a warning that previously separate genetic hemispheres had now been bridged and that East Asia viruses have arrived in the United States.[151] In its early stages the new virus caused very few clinical symptoms, but it quickly evolved more lethal genotypes. By January 2002 a particularly virulent strain appeared on a San Diego farm and spread to other local poultry ranches; infected hens from Southern California were then shipped to Turlock in the Central Valley. A major poultry processing center, Turlock became the hub of an explosive epidemic. As a study published by the Institute of Medicine explains: "Millions of birds shedding viruses traveling in trucks easily spread the infection to farms along the route. That is when the Turlock region, which is bound by three major roads, became known as the Triangle of Doom: a bird couldn't enter the region without becoming infected with H6N2. Tens of millions of birds in California became infected with this H6N2 virus during a four-month period beginning in March 2002."[152]

This massive epidemic—in contrast to the HPAI outbreak in Holland—was largely invisible. From the very beginning, growers used only their own veterinarians and did not release the diagnoses, "not to the state or to other potentially affected states, not to the OIE, not even to neighboring farms, who might have better protected their flocks from infection had they known about it." The emergence of this so-called "Triangle of Doom" was also kept quiet "by corporate decision-makers who feared that consumer demand would plummet if the public knew they were buying infected meat and eggs."[153] As with the SARS outbreak in China the following year, economic interests trumped any concern for public health.

But what, exactly, is the human risk from H6N2? Carol Cardona, a University of California veterinary scientist, emphasizes that LPAI viruses all have the "potential to donate genetic material to potential pandemic strains. The interaction of animal agriculture and the public is complex and dynamic and we do not fully understand the risks associated with various types of contacts between humans and birds."[154] Indeed, many researchers feel that the official distinction between LPAI and HPAI outbreaks is scientifically unsustainable and should not be allowed to dictate different levels of surveillance and response.[155] It is also imperative that agribusiness's bottom line not be allowed to supersede the global priorities of pandemic surveillance and human biosecurity. Amongst the influenzas increasingly seen in the North American poultry industry are H5 and H7 subtypes that display a disturbing tendency to rapidly evolve from LPAIs to HPAIs (Table 7.2). The full danger of not taking LPAIs seriously

Table 7.2.
H5 and H7 (LPAI) Outbreaks in the USA Since 1997[156]

1997	H7N3	Utah
1997–98	H7N2	Pennsylvania
2000	H7N2	Florida
2001	H7N2	Pennsylvania, Maryland, Connecticut
2002	H7N2	Shenandoah Valley, New York, New Jersey
2002	H5N3	Texas
2002	H5N2	New York, Maine, California
2002	H5N8	New York
2002	H5N1	Michigan
2003	H7N2	Connecticut, Rhode Island
2003	H7N2	Human infection in New York
2004	*H5N2*	*Texas (HPAI)*
2004	H7N2	Maryland, Delaware, New Jersey

as human health threats was demonstrated in British Columbia's Fraser Valley in February to May 2004.

In early February of 2004 chickens starting dying on a farm in Abbotsford, east of Vancouver. Authorities classified it as an H7N3 LPAI outbreak and denied rumors that several workers had developed flu symptoms. Canadian Food Inspection Agency officials also withheld information about possible human infection from the provincial Centre for Disease Control, an omission (according to the latter agency) that "could have had severe consequences."[157] The agricultural agents attempted to contain the outbreak within a five-kilometer hot zone, but the virus rapidly mutated to a highly deadly HPAI form, killing whole flocks. (Sequencing later confirmed that a mutation in the hemagglutinin that made it more promiscuously cleavable by host proteases was probably responsible for H7N3's enhanced ability to replicate systemically.)[158] As the epidemic approached the outskirts of Vancouver, the Canadian Food Inspection Agency ordered British Columbia to slaughter the Fraser Valley's entire domestic bird population.

Several dozen workers involved in the gassing and incineration of the 19 million chickens subsequently developed conjunctivitis and/or flu-like symptoms; two definite H7N3 cases were confirmed but the victims were infected by different strains, evidence that the virus was evolving at very high speed.[159] There was also considerable controversy about the disposal of infected chicken excrement after expert testimony that the virus might survive for as long as three months in manure. Although government spokespeople reassured the public that H7 viruses were "quite mild" and not remotely in the same league as the Asian H5N1, Canadian microbiologists warned that H7's "lower virulence should not be inferred to indicate lower pandemic potential since subclinical or mild infections may have greater opportunity through surreptitious spread to reassort, and through mutation, to become more virulent."[160]

The provincial government's management of the outbreak was a fiasco, as even British Columbia's Minister of Agriculture, Food, and Fisheries John van Dongen conceded.[161] Simultaneous epidemics in February 2004 of highly pathogenic H5N2 in Gonzales County, Texas, and LPAI H7N2 in farms in Pennsylvania and in live bird markets in New Jersey only increased the scientific pressure on U.S. and Canadian agricultural authorities to reclassify *all* H5 and H7 outbreaks as HPAI and to expand their respective federal commitments to bird flu surveillance and intervention. The bottom line: world public health cannot afford any holes or blind spots in the pandemic early warning system. As Robert Webster has long advocated, the human-animal interface needs comprehensive monitoring, with local public-health officials around the world supplied with a suitable kit of reagents to allow them to swiftly identify any influenza subtype.[162] The chief lesson taught by the successive poultry epidemics in the Netherlands, California, and British Columbia is that, with avian influenza, the local is always global.

8

Plague and Profit

At the center of the meltdown in Asia's vast
poultry industry is a 61-year-old multi-billionaire
called Dhanin Chearavanont.[163]

Jasper Becker

All of today's tens of billions of highly engineered factory chickens are descended from red jungle fowl that still roam wild in forest regions of Thailand and Vietnam. Using mitochondrial DNA analysis, Japanese researchers in 1994 demonstrated that chickens were domesticated in the area of present-day Thailand more than 8,000 years ago.[164] The chicken, along with the pig and the buffalo, subsequently became the basis of agrarian culture throughout Southeast Asia. Chickens are likewise the bottom line of Asia's largest and most powerful agricultural-export conglomerate, Bangkok-based Charoen Pokphand. CP, as it is universally known, figures centrally in the story of H5N1's terrifying return in the winter of 2003–4 and the unprecedented HPAI epidemic that threatens to become a global human and ecological cataclysm.

Founded by the immigrant Chia brothers from Guangdong, CP was a rice-seed distributor in Bangkok's Chinatown until Chia Ek Chow, the youngest of four sons, took over the business in 1964. In the face of growing intolerance toward the Chinese diaspora throughout Southeast Asia, he changed his name to Dhanin Chearavanont and reoriented the company to chicken breeding and broiler farming. Impressed by the success of U.S. companies in transforming poultry raising into a streamlined industrial process more closely resembling chemical manufacture than traditional agriculture, Chearavanont formed two successive strategic partnerships with American companies and quickly became Asia's leading apostle of Tyson-style intensive farming and vertical integration. In 1973 Chearavanont opened Thailand's first modern poultry slaughterhouse and began exporting to Japan. CP's major competitors, the Bangkok Livestock Trading Company and Saha Farms, were forced to keep pace with Chearavanont's innovations, which included organizing networks of contract farms and building modern export processing plants.

By the mid-1990s, Thailand (which had adopted CP's corporate slogan, "Kitchen of the World,") had the most corporatized livestock industry in Asia. CP and a handful of other vertically-integrated exporters controlled 80 percent of production, with chicken farming concentrated in a dense, polluted belt 60 to 150 kilometers outside Bangkok.[165] With 100,000 employees across Asia, CP boasts that its agro-industrial empire is "fully integrated horizontally and vertically. Operations take in animal feed production, breeders, farming systems, meat processing, food production and its very successful value-added products." CP also has promoted the spectacular rise of Western-style fast foods in Asia through the sourcing, or in the case of China, the direct ownership of myriad Kentucky Fried Chicken franchises.[166]

For Chearavanont and other "integrators," economies of scale in a booming export environment have produced fabulous profits, but for CP's 10,000 contract farmers, as well as for hundreds of thousands of backyard poultry producers, the situation is radically different. As journalist Isabelle Delforge points out: "With contract farming, large companies control the whole production process: they lend money to the farmers, they sell them chicks, feed and medicine, and they have the right to buy the whole production. But usually the company is not committed to buy the chickens if the demand is low. Contract farmers bear all the risks related to production and become extremely dependent on demand from the world market. They become factory workers in their own field." Companies like CP, an organic farmer told Delforge, "destroy small farmers with false promises."[167] For the majority of Thai farmers, the Livestock Revolution has meant soaring indebtedness, loss of independence, and the continued migration of their daughters to Bangkok's sweatshops and brothels.

While Thailand's chickens (and later, pigs and prawns) have made Chearavanont a billionaire and, according to business magazines, one of the twenty most powerful businessmen in Asia, his central ambition has always been to honor his father's dream of bringing the Livestock Revolution—in the form of large-scale agro-industrial capitalism—back to China. Thanks to astute politicking and powerful Guangdong connections, CP was literally the first multinational investor to step foot inside Deng Xiaoping's "Open Door" in 1979 (CP's foreign business license in Shenzhen was number 001). CP, by itself or in alliances with other capital groups, has subsequently invested billions in the PRC. In addition to holding a diversified portfolio of hotels, shopping malls, fast-food franchises (including Kentucky Fried Chicken), telecommunications, and restaurants, it has built more than one hundred feed mills and poultry-processing plants throughout China in an attempt to forestall both foreign competitors (Tyson Foods, above all) and local upstarts in the world's most dynamic market for chicken products.[168] (During the 1990s, as global poultry output surpassed that of beef, China doubled its share of total world consumption—from less than 8 percent to more than 17 percent—and displaced the United States as the largest consumer.)[169]

CP's explosive growth in Thailand and China, as well as its expanding operations in eighteen other countries, has required massive amounts of political grease. In 1996, for example, Chearavanont made an illegal $250,000 donation to the Democratic National Committee in the United States which backfired, causing bad publicity for both CP and the Clinton administration when fundraiser John Huang was indicted. The right-wing *American Spectator* pointed to CP's alliance with a leading Chinese weapon maker and implied that it was one of the "front companies for communist China" that had been "buying up (and spying on) the United States." But the magazine neglected to mention that a few months earlier, Neil Bush, George W.'s brother, had formed a joint venture company with Chearavanont.[170] Indeed, as Dan Moldea and David Corn would later detail in the *Nation*, both the Bush family and the Carlyle Group—the private investment fund used by the family and other leading Republicans to turn insider access into gold— have long-standing and intimate business relations with CP. Former president George H.W. Bush, for example, was reportedly paid $250,000 by CP to lobby Asian and American leaders on its behalf.[171]

Chearavanont also acquired equity in the Thai state in 2001 with the appointment of his son-in-law Wattana Muangsuk as Deputy Commerce Minister. The cell-phone billionaire Thaksin Shinawatra—Siam's answer to Italy's Silvio Berlusconi—won the presidency that year with a lurid populist campaign. Thaksin's political party is called Thai Rak Thai, or "Thai Loves Thai," and he promised debt relief, cheap medical care, and a tough crack-down on drug dealers (2,500 of whom, indeed, were promptly murdered by police death squads). In reality, explains economist Pasuk Phongpaichit, "His ascendency signifies a new consolation of big business and politics. Whereas the business people who have dominated Thai politics since parliament became significant in the 1980s used to be mostly provincial figures of only moderate wealth, Thaksin's government is controlled by the biggest Bangkok business groups to have survived the 1997 crisis."[172] On the eve of the plague, in other words, Thailand was governed by a crony coalition of the telecommunications and livestock industries.

The return of avian influenza was shrouded in rumor, denial, and conspiracy during the fall of 2003. The epidemic actually began much earlier (Indonesia later conceded that H5N1 had been detected in August), but Chinese officials denied reports in the Hong Kong *Standard* that "farms throughout China [had] suffered from avian flu for several years."[173] They also scorned rumors that there was a massive outbreak among ducks in Guangxi Province, bordering Vietnam, and likewise dismissed as Taiwanese propaganda the warning from Taipei that its animal inspectors in December had found H5N1 in wild ducks smuggled from Fujian, the province that was the likely source of the virus that killed two in early 2003.[174]

In January 2004 the British magazine *New Scientist,* interviewing leading flu researchers off the record, created a small tempest with claims that the outbreak was the result of a clandestine and misguided vaccination campaign ("an uncontrolled experiment in viral evolution") by poultry producers in south China after the 1997 crisis in Hong Kong. By using an inactivated virus to immunize their chickens, Chinese growers had actually accelerated the evolution of an H5N1 superstrain— genotype Z (GenZ)—that quickly became endemic but asymptomatic in domestic ducks. From this stable reservoir, it began to spread to other species via direct contact, poultry smuggling, and possibly by wild bird migration. According to the *New Scientist,* "a combination of official cover-up and questionable farming practices allowed it to turn into the epidemic now under way."[175]

But Chinese authorities were not the only ones concealing the epidemic. In early November 2003, chickens started dying on farms across Thailand. As one farmer described it: "Their bodies began shaking; it was if they were suffocating, and thick saliva started coming out their mouths. We tried to give the hens herbs to make them better, but it made no difference. The faces then went dark green and black, and then they died."[176] Although a veterinary scientist at Bangkok's Chulalongkorn University warned that he found H5N1 in several dead chickens, he was ignored by Thailand's Livestock Department. ("All the academics and experts," an opposition senator would later allege, "had to shut up due to political interference.") Likewise, when a worried farmer showed the carcasses of his dead flock to an official, he was told that the birds had died "without any medical cause."[177]

Strangely, in the midst of all these bird deaths, the corporate chicken-processing plants were working overtime. As angry trade unionists at one factory just outside the capital told the *Bangkok Post* after the scandal broke: "Before November we were processing about 90,000 chickens a day. But from November to 23 January, we had to kill about 130,000 daily. It's our job to cut the birds up. It was obvious they were ill: their organs were swollen. We didn't know what the disease was, but we understood that the management was rushing to process the chickens before getting any veterinary inspection. We stopped eating [chicken] in October."[178]

The wall of official silence across Asia was breached in December when chickens started dying en masse on a farm near Seoul. Korean agricultural officials were stunned to discover H5N1, but, in contrast to their counterparts in China and Thailand, they promptly notified the Office International des Epizooties (OIE); a week later, South Korea announced a massive cull after new infections were identified in chicken and duck flocks in five provinces. Meanwhile children, not just chickens, had been dying mysteriously in Vietnam; just before the New Year, one of the CDC's influenza experts in Atlanta received a worried email from a virologist in Hanoi which described patients suffering from symptoms of viral pneumonia and acute respiratory distress syndrome (ARDS), which had caused the death of many of the 1918 pandemic's victims.

The Hanoi doctor and her colleagues were unaware that their own agriculture bureaucracy had been concealing, at least since October, evidence of a sporadic H5N1 epidemic among poultry.[179] On 5 January 2004, following the deaths of several more people, Vietnamese public-health officers urgently requested help from the WHO, whose regional office in Manila also soon heard rumors as well of Vietnam's HPAI outbreak; a few days later Hong Kong experts confirmed that the Frankenstein GenZ had been found in forensic samples from three of the dead children in Hanoi. Simultaneously, Vietnam officially acknowledged an avian flu epidemic in two provinces and Japan announced the discovery of H5N1 among hens in Yamaguchi prefecture. (The outbreak in western Japan had originally been concealed by poultry company officials—one of whom later committed suicide—and only came to light thanks to an anonymous tip-off from a company employee.)[180]

The WHO and its veterinary counterpart, the OIE, as well as the UN Food and Agricultural Organization (FAO), were horrified to realize that bureaucrats and agribusiness spokespeople had for months been covering up an avian flu epidemic of continental scope. (In impeccable, understated bureaucratese, FAO Director-General Jacques Diouf observed that "the lack of timely reporting of infection to the national competent authorities, OIE and other international bodies has contributed to the scale of the problem.")[181] Facing an increasingly cynical world press, it became almost impossible for the international agencies to accept the reassurances that continued to flow from Chinese and Thai ministries—the Chinese, in particular, seemed to have reverted to the Orwellian culture of secrecy and deception previously associated with the Jiang Zemin camp. When another mystery respiratory infection swept Guangdong in January 2004, officials dismissed it (shades of SARS) as the bacterium *Chlamydia pneumoniae* and refused to let the WHO investigate on the spot. (A skeptical Chinese researcher told *Nature*: "But that can't be the whole story. From a clinical standpoint, it seems to be related to a virus, and we cannot rule out the bird flu.")[182]

In Thailand, meanwhile, lies were being manufactured almost as fast as sick chickens were being slaughtered and shipped to overseas markets. Deputy Minister of Agriculture Newin Chidchob talked nonchalantly about a few cases of "avian cholera," while Prime Minister Thaksin and his ministers, to assuage a nervous public, "devoured a big feast of deliciously cooked, Thai-style chicken dishes in a nationwide television broadcast."[183] CP senior executive Sarasin Viraphol assured reporters that, although the company would not allow the press to inspect its plants, avian flu was completely absent in Thailand. In fact, as the Bangkok press later reported, the government had been colluding with CP and the other giant poultry producers to conceal the epidemic by paying contract farmers with infected flocks to keep quiet; official deceit gave the big exporters several months to process and sell diseased inventory as well as to disinfect their plants and institute isolation procedures in their battery warehouses. Small producers, however, were left alone to bear the brunt of the epidemic's human and economic costs.[184]

Finally, in late January, with two young farm boys critically ill from influenza, the Thai parliamentary opposition, led by maverick senator Nirum Phitakwatchara, was able to force Prime Minister Thaksin Shinawatra to admit that H5N1 was, in fact, ravaging the poultry belt. His staff immediately off-loaded responsibility for official mendacity onto lowly provincial officials. "What looks like a cover-up," Thaksin's spokesman deadpanned, "was a misinterpretation of procedures. The most appropriate word is 'screw-up.' Some agencies screwed up. We found there was lots of confusion about the kinds of information that needed to be reported upstairs."[185]

Small producers, in response, screamed that "by denying the facts, the government was helping out the major operators, but in the end it's us small farmers who are suffering."[186] A Bangkok newspaper contrasted the fate of big and small poultry producers in Sukhothai province. The commercial growers "integrated" by CP and other conglomerates were notified about the epidemic in December and were provided with antiviral vaccines by livestock officials, and thus their inventories were saved. But small holders were kept in the dark about the disease, and as a result most of their chickens perished as did one peasant's teenage son. "If we had at least known about the disease," Laweng Boonrod told the press, "I would not have allowed my son to go close to my sick chickens and he would not have died."[187]

The main importers of Thai poultry were also furious at the elaborate deception, none more so than EU Health Commissioner, David Byrne, who had just returned to Brussels with Prime Minister Thaksin's personal assurance that Thailand was free of avian flu. Byrne told the press that he "felt dishonored."[188] The EU, Japan, and South Korea promptly embargoed poultry imports from Thailand, while the Bush administration, grateful for Thaksin's support of U.S. interventions in Afghanistan and Iraq, avoided public criticism of the cover-up.

CP's stock immediately fell by an eighth, and the ground shook. ("In Thailand," writes Isabelle Delforge, "when CP sneezes, the whole business community catches cold—or flu.")[189] Dhanin Chearavanont, however, was surprisingly upbeat and urged Thais to "turn the crisis into opportunity." Another CP executive promised that "changes resulting from the crisis would benefit the Thai chicken industry in the long term as well as help it recover from the current difficulties." The plague, in other words, might rationalize poultry production. But opportunities and benefits for whom? The government quickly unveiled a sweeping plan to complete the modernization of the Thai poultry industry by culling small-scale, open-air flocks and requiring their operators to build new industrial poultry houses; only those farmers who fully complied with the plan would be eligible for compensation for their dead chickens.

Thailand's agrarian populists, including senator and agricultural economist Chirmsak Pinthong, promptly denounced the government's plan as another cunning move by Chearavanont to force the small operators into the extinction or turn them into serfs of CP.* "The government is regulating small chicken raisers in such a way that it benefits the big conglomerates."[190] Small holders complained that government compensation for their dead chickens was only a fraction of what CP and others were charging them to restock their flocks. There was also evidence that the poultry cull was being used to strengthen the corporations. "When the avian flu was detected," writes Delforge and a Thai colleague, "a red zone was cleared around the farm and all the poultry in the zone were killed to prevent the spread of the disease. However, some farmers reported dead chickens but no red zone was declared around their property. They suspected the authorities of

---

* An Internet lunatic fringe, American not Thai, maintains that both CP and Tyson are engaged in clandestine biowarfare against small-scale producers and that H5N1 may be their designer weapon. The impetus for this stupidity seems to be both corporations' former support for ex-President Bill Clinton.

protecting neighboring industrial farms or owners of highly valuable fighting cocks."[191]

He Changchui, FAO Assistant Director-General and Regional Representative for Asia and the Pacific, indirectly criticized the giant producers by stressing the role of "high densities of humans and animals . . . [in] creating new pathways for disease transmission through inappropriate waste disposal, direct contact or through airborne transmission." He urged a "substantial restructuring" of poultry production along lines that favored the poor, protected the environment, and compensated the small producers affected by the outbreak.[192] The Thaksin government, however, uncritically embraced Chearavanont's contention that avian flu's spread was due to the small producers and their "backward" open-air chicken flocks. CP claimed that its industrialized, enclosed farming system was virtually impregnable to viral outbreaks and epidemics.

While it is true that Southeast Asia's traditional backyard chicken flocks offer myriad opportunities for infectious interchange between different species of poultry and wild birds, the huge chicken factories (50,000 birds per two-story structure) maximize the accumulation of viral load and subsequent antigenic drift. Indeed, disease ecologists believe that "a high density of smallholders surrounding intensive or industrial units" creates "a particularly risky situation."[193] In an epidemiological sense, the outdoor flocks are the fuse, and the dense factory populations, the explosive charge. Moreover, as Delforge emphasizes in one of her exemplary reports, CP's factory farms have themselves been identified as vectors of the epidemic: "In Vietnam, the current chicken flu outbreak infected a large closed farm owned by CP." As *Vietnam News* reported on 4 February 2004,

"The army has been mobilized to kill 117,000 birds on the biggest farm in Ha Tay province, owned by the Thai Charoen Pokphand Company."[194]

Once the Thais had publicly acknowledged their outbreak, the other major deceivers—Indonesia and China—were forced to play show-and-tell as well. The scandal of Indonesia's 2 February confession that the government had been concealing knowledge of an H5N1 outbreak since late August was compounded by Agriculture Minister Bungaran Saragih's extraordinary explanation that they had withheld information because "we did not want to cause unnecessary losses through a hasty decision."[195] The minister also asserted that the strain of H5N1 circulating in eighty districts from Sumatra to Kalimantan and West Timor, which had already killed 15 million chickens, was different from the virus in Vietnam and posed no threat to humans—a claim dismissed as nonsense by scientists.

Chinese officials managed to be even more arrogant and egregious in their attempt to save face than their Indonesian counterpart. In the first week of February they grudgingly doled out in bits and pieces the admission that H5N1 was raging in no fewer than twelve provinces and cities, including Guanxi, Guangdong, and even metropolitan Shanghai. Ten days later, Chen Kaizhi, a top official in Guangzhou, demonstrated the stunning scientific ignorance of senior bureaucrats like himself in a speech to the Guangdong People's Congress: "This disease is hundreds of years old and it can be prevented and treated. Vaccines are effective. No humans have been infected, so why this uproar?" Chen went on to contrast the hysteria of Hong Kong health officials, the WHO and other "outsiders" with traditional folk wisdom. "In the past when life was hard, we hoped for a disease among our chickens so that we got to eat chicken. When a chicken at home dropped its head, we said, 'good, now we get to eat chicken.' Now we are so advanced that people are not allowed to eat diseased chicken."[196]

Chen, of course, ignored the fact that, thanks to the cover-ups in Guangdong and elsewhere, thousands of people had consumed diseased chicken products. Meanwhile, the Hong Kong media that had earlier reported suspected cases in the PRC or now dared to criticize the ignorance of officials like Chen were threatened with legal action under the same infamous mainland statute that had been used to suppress reportage of SARS a year earlier.

While observers speculated about what had happened to the short-lived reign of scientific and medical "transparency" in China, the OIE and WHO were desperately worried about the haphazard, and, in some cases, perfunctory character of the poultry culls that were Asia's only hope of containing the H5N1

Table 8.1.
Covering-up the Epidemic

Country	Official Admission	Actual Onset
S. Korea	12/12/03	
Vietnam	1/8/04	10/03
Japan	1/12/04	
Thailand	1/23/04	11/03
Cambodia	1/24/04	
China	1/27/04	early 03
Laos	1/27/04	
Indonesia	2/2/04	8/03

catastrophe. In Thailand, where prisoners were mobilized under army supervision to bury millions of chickens alive, the flocks of small producers, as we have seen, were dutifully massacred, while corporate chickens received special treatment. Activists charged that "workers and consumers' health clearly comes after exporters' wealth," and the WHO scolded the government for its lackadaisical attitude toward protecting farmers and cullers from infection. Thai authorities also wasted valuable time in the needless slaughter of wild birds and urban pigeons after Prime Minister Thaksin, in characteristic xenophobic fashion, blamed "foreign" wildfowl for starting the epidemic.[197]

The government of Vietnam, previously praised by the WHO for its competent handling of the SARS outbreak, was altogether more cooperative, but the country's poverty and the dispersed character of its largely backyard poultry industry posed huge obstacles to creating effective viral firebreaks. Poor farmers suppressed news of infections and concealed valuable birds such as fighting cocks; in addition, in face of rising anger in the countryside, the government was reluctant to extend the radius of culls around sick flocks beyond one half kilometer—the WHO recommended three kilometers—or to exterminate the domestic ducks that were the infection's probable reservoir. Similarly, the disinfection of farms and the disposal of contaminated poultry manure were Sisyphean tasks that always risked further transmission of the virus, typically via the boots or clothing of cleanup workers. No sooner was an outbreak suppressed in one part of the country than another appeared in a different province. Small children, who frequently played outside with chickens and ducks and were constantly exposed to poultry waste, were particularly vulnerable to these seemingly ineradicable village outbreaks.[198]

Indonesian President Megawati Sukarnoputri, meanwhile, balked at the task of killing millions of chickens, and so her government initially proposed a vaccination campaign instead. After angry protests from the rest of the ASEAN bloc, Indonesia finally agreed to slaughter birds, but with a half-heartedness that reassured few critics. The WHO, however, continued to have the most difficulty with Beijing. "We have repeatedly said there is a brief window of opportunity to act within China," warned a WHO representative at the beginning of February 2004, "This latest news [outbreaks in Hunan and Hubei] strongly suggests that the window is getting smaller with each passing day." Another WHO official told the Associated Press that "mass culling is not taking place at the speed we consider absolutely necessary to contain the virus."[199] *The Lancet*, for its part, warned in February that China's "animal-disease surveillance is as good as absent, a vacuum into which global health might hopelessly and terrifyingly fall."[200] When leading influenza expert Robert Webster suggested in another *Lancet* article that the time had come to consider closing down China's live-animal markets, he was ignored.[201]

February was, indeed, a terrifying month, with new human victims in Vietnam and Thailand and further avian outbreaks in China and Indonesia. WHO teams, reinforced with a cadre of top experts from American, European, and Japanese laboratories, struggled with the imminent possibility of a global pandemic against which the world would have little protection. An experimental vaccine developed in 1997 was ineffective against GenZ, which was also resistant to amantadine, the cheapest and most common antiviral. (Hong Kong researchers feared this was further evidence of human tampering in the evolution of H5N1 and urged an investigation of chicken feed to test for amantadine-like molecules.)[202]

Most disturbingly, the new strain was more lethal than any influenza in scientific experience. In the course of the viral pneumonia it engendered, GenZ was stunningly adept at inducing deadly "cytokine storms" in which victims' own berserk immune systems destroyed their lungs and other organs; two-thirds of GenZ's victims (twenty-two out of thirty-three) had died by 9 March, and, unlike its 1997 cousin, it relished toddlers and teenagers as well as adults.[203] With each passing day, scientists feared they would meet its reassortant offspring, ready to conquer the world, but despite their repeated warnings only one country—Canada—had undertaken truly serious preparations to meet the pandemic threat.[204] In the meantime, only the dismal, dirty work of the slaughter—some 120 million chickens were eventually buried alive, burnt to death, electrocuted, or gassed—offered any hope of preventing a fatal rendezvous between a nightmare virus and a vulnerable humanity.

Then in mid-March, the plague suddenly seemed to relent. The last deaths were a twelve-year-old in Vietnam, who passed away on 15 March after a long struggle, and a poultry worker in Thailand who died the following day. On 16 March, China announced that it had eradicated the virus in all forty-nine hot zones; this triumphalist statement alarmed the FAO and the OIE, who cautioned against premature declarations of victory—the international protocol was to carefully monitor flocks for six months before ruling that a region or nation was free of avian influenza. The international agencies warned that the crisis was not over, and they warned countries not to restock poultry until they had adequate surveillance and biosecurity in place.[205]

Nonetheless, Vietnam followed China's example on 30 March and declared the outbreak over.

Thailand also intimated that it was making splendid progress and would soon join the ranks of the victors. As CP shares began to climb out of the gutter and the Thaksin regime lobbied Europe and Japan to re-admit Thai chicken products, the attention of the international influenza community shifted to the alarming H7 outbreak in British Columbia. Somehow, despite the cover-ups, official lies, and months of lost ground, and despite the bungled culls and the gaping holes in the influenza surveillance network, the great chicken slaughter nevertheless seemed to have turned the tide. The WHO's warnings about an imminent pandemic seemed less urgent, and the more optimistic, especially the politicians and exporters, thought they had defeated H5N1. But alas, the virus had simply taken a brief vacation.

9

Edge of the Abyss

Pandemic? Very, very likely.[206]
WHO regional director for Asia

The economic impact of the avian flu epidemic on the Southeast Asian countryside was profound. Thousands of small chicken farmers were bankrupted and forced out of business, thus yielding ground, as Chearavanont had urged, to the corporate operators. Meanwhile, the unprecedented market turbulence unleashed by the H5 epidemic in Asia, followed by the H7 outbreaks in North America, encouraged the big poultry producers to poach one another's customers. In the United States, giants like Tyson and Pilgrim's Pride were "already reaping some benefits from the bird flu virus" in late January as they rushed exports to replace the quarantined Thai supply. Jim Summer, president of the Poultry and Egg Export Council, told reporters that the avian flu "is going to have an unbelievable impact on the poultry industry" and boasted of a surge in hiring by U.S. companies. CP, meanwhile, exploited its own disaster by increasing exports from plants in Taiwan and other nonembargoed countries to take advantage of the sharp rise in chicken prices. To offset current and future EU import controls, Chearavanont also announced an ambitious expansion of poultry operations in

Romania, Russia, and Ukraine, and he reassured his shareholders that they would soon reap profit from the influenza-driven restructuring of global chicken production.[207]

All of this cheery news from the giant chicken producers was of little solace to the researchers struggling to understand the spectacular menace of H5N1 GenZ. An extraordinary research consortium combining the resources of Robert Webster's St. Jude Hospital group, the veteran team from the University of Hong Kong, and local experts from across Asia had been working feverishly to unravel the genealogy and molecular structure of the 2003–4 strain. To achieve a panoramic view of its evolution, they sequenced and compared the genomes of hundreds of viral samples obtained from human victims and poultry. Their findings were disturbing.

In a letter to *Nature* in July 2004, they warned the virus's erstwhile conquerors that, in fact, avian flu—now comfortably ensconced among asymptomatic domestic ducks—was almost ineradicable. "H5N1 is now endemic in poultry in Asia and has gained an entrenched ecological niche from which to present a long-term pandemic threat to humans." Moreover, its sudden retreat in March might have had more to do with influenza's seasonal cycle than with the mass murder of chickens: "Since 2001, H5N1 viruses have continued to circulate in mainland China with a seasonal pattern, peaking from October to March, when the mean temperature is below 20 centigrade." They also noted that "the timing and distribution of the H5N1 infection in China from 2001 onwards coincides with the general period of winter bird migration to southern China: however it is not know whether the H5N1 virus has become established in wild bird populations."[208]

Although they now possessed a detailed map of the structure of GenZ—each protein had been analysed to the last amino acid group—they were still baffled by its functional organization: they had, so to speak, a splendid view of the wiring, but only a fragmentary concept of its purpose. They knew that GenZ, the sole survivor of a marathon competition between more than a dozen H5N1 genotypes, was a superfit strain, and was evolving rapidly as it passed back and forth between different populations and species. (Other studies would show that GenZ was far more environmentally stable than the 1997 strain and that it was becoming progressively more skillful in infecting mammals.)[209] They also knew that natural selection, horrifyingly, seemed to favor increased virulence in humans, but they were unable to nail down the molecular determinants of the human infections in Vietnam and Thailand or, for that matter, explain why H5N1 had not yet acquired pandemic transmissibility. The researchers noted potentially synergistic mutations at strategic sites in the H5 molecule as well as in proteins (PB2 and NSI) involved with replication and immune suppression, but they refrained from speculating how these variations were choreographed in avian or human infections.[210]

Gen Z, in other words, was not giving away any secrets. Although leading researchers would presumably all concur with evolutionary biologist Simon Levin that "influenza presents a [evolutionary] system that is second to none in terms of complexity," there had been considerable optimism that a "smoking gun" of some kind would emerge from the high-powered research teams doing parallel work on H5N2 and the resurrected genome of the 1918 virus—science seemed tantalizingly close to unlocking the secret of why some influenzas were such vicious killers. The team working on recovered fragments of the 1918 genome, led by Jeffery Taubenberger, Ann Reid, and Thomas Fanning at the Armed Forces Institute of Pathology in Maryland, had made breathtaking progress in unraveling the molecular structure of H1N1/1918, but they had failed to resolve the central question of the source of its pathogenicity. Indeed, their research to date has only reframed the essential mysteries of the great pandemic, offering "no definite clue to [its] exceptional virulence," while casting doubt on the traditional hypothesis that it originated either in swine or ordinary waterfowl.[211]

By the summer of 2004, in other words, the world's elite influenza researchers had reached the sobering consensus that avian influenza would neither go away nor allow itself to be easily understood. ("It's troubling to me," leading CDC researcher Keiji Fukuda confided to the *New York Times* in fall 2004, "that we still don't know much more about this virus than we did in 1997.")[212] Many also had begun to worry that the virus might bypass the textbook requirement to reassort with a human influenza and simply evolve on its own to the pandemic stage by the simple accumulation of a few more mutations. "Mutation during human infection," the WHO had cautioned in April, "is a second mechanism for improving transmissibility; scientists believe that only a small number of mutational changes in the virus may be needed."[213] In August Western scientists were shocked to discover that a team of Chinese virologists from the Harbin Veterinary Research Institute had published a paper in January in which they reported that H5N1 was widespread in swine in southeast China and urged utmost "pandemic preparedness." That such an important report should have passed unnoticed for months by the

WHO and FAO hardly inspired confidence in global influenza surveillance.[214]

Just as researchers feared, GenZ came creeping back at the end of spring, infecting a mixed flock of chickens and waterfowl at a university research farm in Thailand in late May; by July there were widespread outbreaks in Vietnam, central Thailand, and China's Anhui province. Thai officials again responded by blaming foreign birds and ordered crews to exterminate open-bill storks and chop down the trees they nested in. (An ornithologist despaired: "I've never seen anything like it. Birds had become the enemy.")[215] In mid-August veterinary officers discovered Malaysia's first case of H5N1 in a pair of fighting cocks returned from a match in Thailand: troubling evidence that the prized sporting birds were now a vector of infection. Vietnam then shattered hopes with a belated announcement that three people, including two young sisters, had died between 30 July and 3 August in Hau Giang province, southwest of Ho Chi Minh City.[216]

Bad news grew worse in September with human deaths reported in Thailand, the first being a eighteen-year-old game-bird trainer. As they investigated, WHO officials were horrified to find out that it was common practice for the owners of fighting cocks to suck blood and mucous from the beaks of birds injured in a fight. Over the next two weeks an eleven-year-old girl and a thirteen-year-old boy died, while nine other children languished in intensive care. Dr. Shigeru Omi, the WHO's Regional Director for the Western Pacific Region, warned emphatically in mid-September that "unless intensified efforts are made to halt the spread of the virus, a pandemic is very likely to occur."[217] In an oafish attempt to reassure international opinion that his government was on the job, the Director of the Department of Livestock Development, Yukol Limlamthong, emphasized that avian flu outbreaks had been identified in "only 56 locations across 23 provinces . . . not hundreds of spots as in some news reports." The exasperated head of the Public Health Ministry, Dr. Charal Trinwuthipong, promptly blasted Limlamthong's department for its negligence in monitoring and reporting outbreaks: "They've not improved! How damned lousy they were last time, that's how they still are."[218]

While the fur was flying between Thai ministries, simultaneous outbreaks of H5N1 and H3N2 in several districts in Thailand again raised the specter of pandemic reassortment. Despite pleas from leading public-health experts, Prime Minister Thaksin refused to import vaccine from Europe to protect the country's exposed populations. He did, however, robustly defend CP against embarrassing charges by Cambodian farmers that chickens purchased from CP Cambodia Ltd. were the source of a new outbreak in that country.[219] He also proposed to aid the big exporters by bartering their contaminated chicken to Moscow. "When we can't sell in our traditional markets, we need to penetrate new markets by bartering. We can't leave all this chicken in Thailand." He ordered his ambassador in Moscow to offer a mountain of chicken in exchange for Sukol SU-30 fighters for the Thai air force. Vladimir Putin, unsurprisingly, declined to accept the bargain.[220]

All this, however, was just a bizarre prelude to the devastating news revealed to the world by the WHO on 28 September: Pranee Thongchan in Kamphaeng Phet was the first victim of a probable human-to-human transmission of the virus, which she contracted from her mortally ill daughter (see Preface). Although

Klaus Stohr, the former East German veterinarian who was now head of the WHO Global Influenza Program, reassured the public that the case was epidemiologically a "nonsustained, inefficient, dead-end street," CDC scientists were, in fact, frantically sequencing viral samples from the dead mother and daughter to see if GenZ had "mutated significantly—or worse, reassorted with a human flu"—a possible consequence of the government's failure to vaccinate hot-spot populations. In a joint statement, the WHO and FAO warned that avian influenza was now "a crisis of global importance."[221]

Although no human flu genes were found in the viral samples, Pranee's death was an earthquake that thoroughly shook international confidence in Thailand. More than chicken exports were now endangered: tourism, the source of 6 percent of the nation's GDP, was under threat. Prime Minister Thaksin responded with a tantrum in which he blamed the "ignorance" of villagers for the persistence of the outbreak and—music to the ears of corporate poultry producers—threatened to ban farm families from raising fowl in their yards. He melodramatically ordered his ministers to eradicate the flu in a month or lose their heads. And facing charges that livestock authorities were bungling the monitoring of poultry, he called for a million volunteers to search the country for sick chickens. "I want to X-ray every single inch of the country," he told provincial governors. "If we see dead birds during the inspection, we will assume that it's bird flu and start culling in the region. The government will spend any amount of money on the project."[222]

Thaksin's crusade against small farmers and wild birds, however, did not prevent further deaths. Neighbors of nine-year-old Kanda Siluangon, who died in early October, "blamed district and provincial livestock officials, saying they did nothing for one month after being notified of the chicken deaths."[223] A female worker at a chicken-processing plant died a few days later, followed in mid-October by a fourteen-year-old farm girl. The most unexpected victims in October, however, were cats, big and small. As their horrified keepers stood helpless, more than eighty Bengal tigers at the famed Sriracha Tiger Zoo near Bangkok perished in spasms of viral pneumonia. They had been fed raw chicken. Similarly, GenZ was identified in house cats, presumably as a result of their feeding on infected poultry or wild birds. Influenza experts were dismayed because cats had long been considered resistant to all varieties of influenza A. They also discovered that cats could pass the virus to each other, making felines suddenly suspect as significant flu vectors and possible incubators.[224]

Then, on 26 October, Europe was provided with a first-hand demonstration of how comprehensively GenZ was spreading through Southeast Asian fauna after a Thai smuggler was stopped at the Brussels airport; he had two tiny rare eagles hidden in a PVC pipe in his hand luggage. The man was eventually let go, and the birds were put into quarantine. A few days later they tested positive for H5N1, setting off a frantic hunt to identify passengers who might have had inadvertent contact with the smuggler. The veterinarian who was called in to euthanize the little eagles (as well as the four hundred other birds in quarantine at the airport) developed a mild but nonetheless alarming case of conjunctivitis. Belgium's leading influenza expert, Rene Snacken, at the Scientific Institute of Public Health, warned *New Scientist*: "We were very, very lucky. It could have been a bomb for Europe."[225]

A few weeks later, Ken Shortridge, the senior member of the famed Hong Kong team that had battled H5N1 in 1997 and SARS in 2003, told a scientific conference that the increasing interspecies transmission of avian influenza risked something even more profound than a new human pandemic. "If this virus gets into bird life beyond poultry," he warned, "we could wreck the global ecosystem." Eight years of research on H5N1 had convinced him that this cunning little Darwinian demon was capable of ecocide—the wiping out of entire species.[226]

There was no shortage of dismaying visions in the late fall of 2004. When *Newsweek* asked a leading microbiologist whether a pandemic was possible, he replied, "I don't think we completely understand why it hasn't happened already."[227] Indeed, there was broad agreement among researchers that an H5 pandemic was not simply imminent, it was "late." Getting this urgent message across to news media, the nonspecialist medical community, NGOs, and ultimately, to presidents, prime ministers, and kings the world over was the urgent task entrusted to the WHO (in theory, the medical conscience of humanity). It was an uneven and divided effort compromised by undue deference to the interests of powerful states, including China and the United States, which generated some lurid headlines and rhetorical promises but none of the truly decisive action urged by experts on the ground.

In late October, a conference at Cold Spring Harbor on Long Island, sponsored by the Sabin Vaccine Institute, brought WHO authorities, U.S. health officials, and drug manufacturers together to discuss a global vaccine strategy in face of the pandemic threat. This dialogue was resumed in Geneva in mid-November under WHO auspices. A parade of experts complained that "very little action" had been taken to avert pandemic "devastation," and the WHO's Klaus Stohr told delegates, "If we continue as we are now, there will be no vaccine available, let alone antivirals, when the next pandemic starts." He also played to the U.S. obsession with terrorism by urging counties "to raise the profile of pandemic preparedness as a matter of national security."[228] An Aventis-Pasteur executive, however, warned public-health officials that manufacturers were prepared to develop new vaccines only if governments were willing to underwrite the costs of research and guarantee sales. The position of the drug industry, in other words, was "no vaccine" unless broad profit margins were guaranteed. This excluded participation by most poor countries. Apart from South Africa and Brazil, which already produce small quantities of annual flu vaccine, the prospects for a truly "global" vaccine that would be available in the Third World were bleak at best. A third WHO-sponsored meeting in Bangkok at the end of November elicited new pledges from ASEAN health ministers, who promised regional coordination in an intensified fight against the poultry plague; however, no concrete commitments emerged dealing with live-animal markets, vaccine development, or the stockpiling of antivirals.[229]

Many researchers and activists wondered if the WHO was not being too meek in sounding the tocsin. In particular, they worried that WHO's influenza czar, Klaus Stohr, had been deliberately underselling the menace of H5N1 in order to safeguard the organization's credibility in the face of skeptical governments. When asked about possible mortality, Stohr routinely referred to a U.S. CDC study that projected 2 to 7.4 million deaths globally, but CDC health economist Martin Meltzer had derived these figures by extrapolating from the mild 1968

Table 9.1.
How Many Might Die?

1957 mortality	2 million
1968 mortality	0.7 million
1968 extrapolated (Stohr)	2 to 7.4 million
1918 mortality	40 to 100 million
Omi's estimate	7 to 100 million
1918 extrapolated	325 million (maximum)
H5N1 mortality extrapolated	1 billion

pandemic; most influenza experts actually feared that H5N1 could become as deadly as the 1918 virus. Michael Osterholm, the respected director of the Center for Infectious Disease Research and Policy at the University of Minnesota, characterized Stohr's cautious estimates as "rather ridiculous."[230]

Most of the scientific community, therefore, was heartened when the WHO's Shigeru Omi evoked the 1918 precedent when he warned the press on 29 November: "We are talking at least seven million [deaths], but maybe more—10 million, 20 million and the worst case, 100 million." (Omi was still being conservative: an direct extrapolation of maximum 1918 mortality to today's world population would be 325 million dead.) The cat was out of the bag, and top experts, like Malik Peiris at the University of Hong Kong, rushed to defend Omi's figures as "consistent with current research." Scotland's *Sunday Herald*, moreover, in mid-December printed frightening excerpts from a leaked UK government study that projected a near-breakdown of British society during a pandemic. "A minimum of 25 percent of the population will become ill over each six- to eight-week period. . . . Mortality is likely to be high—estimated at 1 percent of the total population."

The WHO ultimately bowed to majority opinion and, over Stohr's objections, revised his previous estimates as "a best-case scenario"; 50 million dead was now officially the "worst case." Yet a few epidemiologists think even 50 million dead is wishful thinking. Extrapolating from the current lethality of GenZ rather than from 1918 mortality (i.e., 72 percent versus 2.5 percent), they reminded officials that the true worst-case scenario, in fact, was more in the range of *1 billion* deaths.[231]

10

Homeland Insecurity

*Regardless of human endeavors, nature's
on-going experiments with H5N1 influenza in
Asia and H7N7 in Europe may be the greatest
bioterror threat of all.*[232]

Richard Webby and Robert Webster

On 3 December 2004, U.S. Secretary of Health and Human Services (HHS) Tommy Thompson held a press conference to announce his resignation. His turbulent, heavy-handed reign had alienated most of the leading disease researchers at the National Institutes of Health (NIH) and elsewhere. "I don't think," one senior scientist told *Nature*, "you're going to find very many people at the NIH who are doing anything but jumping for joy."[233] Yet his tenure ended with a note of frankness rare in the Bush era. Unlike the previous seven cabinet members purged in the President Bush's postelection housecleaning, Thompson, according to the *New York Times*, "gave candid, unexpected answers to questions posed to him." He complained, for instance, that Congress, ever solicitous of the pharmaceutical industry, had refused to give him authority to negotiate lower prices for Medicare prescriptions. He also agreed with FDA critics that an independent watchdog of the agency was needed in the wake of scandals about the safety of Vioxx and other drugs. "Asked what worried him most, Mr. Thompson cited the threat of a human flu pandemic. . . . 'This is a really huge bomb that could adversely impact on the health of the world,' killing 30 million to 70 million people, he said."[234]

The secretary, of course, spoke with the authority of someone with access to the best medical intelligence in the world, but reporters were undoubtedly surprised that Thompson was so alarmed about a peril that his department with its $543 billion annual budget—a quarter of the federal total—had done so little to address. In the last fiscal year, for example, Thompson had allocated more funds to "abstinence education" than to the development of an avian influenza vaccine that might save millions of lives.[235] This is but one example of the way that all Americans, but especially children, the elderly, and the uninsured, have been placed in harm's way by the Bush regime's bizarre skewing of public-health priorities. On Thompson's watch, HHS and the Pentagon spent $14.5 billion to safeguard national security against largely hypothetical biological threats like smallpox and anthrax, even as they pursued a penny-pinching strategy to deal with the most dangerous and likely "bioterrorist": avian influenza. The administration's lackadaisical response to the pandemic threat (despite Secretary Thompson's personal anxiety) is only the tip of the iceberg. Over the last generation, writes *Lancet* editor Richard Horton, "The U.S. public-health system has been slowly and quietly falling apart."[236]

Under Democrats as well as Republicans, Washington has looked the other way as local health departments have lost funding and crucial hospital surge capacity has been eroded in the wake of the HMO revolution. (A sobering 2004 Government

Accounting Office [GAO] report confirmed that "no state is fully prepared to respond to a major public-health threat.")[237] The federal government also has refused to address the growing lack of new vaccines and antibiotics caused by the pharmaceutical industry's withdrawal from sectors judged to be insufficiently profitable; moreover, revolutionary breakthroughs in vaccine design and manufacturing technology have languished due to lack of sponsorship by either the government or the drug industry.

As discussed in an earlier chapter, the so-called "fiasco" of the swine flu vaccine in 1977 was used as an excuse by the Reagan administration to discard the Carter–Califano policy of gradually widening the scope of annual influenza vaccinations. Reagan-era medical priorities were cancer and heart disease— "middle-class" health issues with broad electoral resonance— rather than infectious disease or community-based medicine; as a consequence, savage federal cutbacks in the early 1980s led the Institute of Medicine to warn in 1987 that the United States was ill-prepared to face the threat of emergent diseases. The Institute declared: "The decline in preparedness and effectiveness of the nation's first-line medical defense systems can be traced to these ill advised budget cuts which forced the termination of essential and research and training programs."[238] A year later, with AIDS raging in big American cities and infectious disease mortality increasing by nearly 5 percent annually, Institute authors added, "We have let down our public health guard as a nation and the health of the public is unnecessarily threatened as a result." Yet another Institute of Medicine report in 1992, authored by Joshua Lederberg and Robert Shope, contrasted the breakdown of the public-health infrastructure with the radical changes in disease ecology being wrought by globalization.[239]

There was great hope that the Clinton administration with its strategic focus on health-care reform would finally re-arm the country to adequately face the new viral perils, but as writer Greg Behrman recounts in his bitter history of how Washington "slept through the global AIDS pandemic," Clinton public-health policy was undermined by the administration's own fetishism of deficit reduction, followed by the Republican capture of Congress in 1994.[240] To her credit, Donna Shalala, Clinton's HHS secretary, did establish a pandemic influenza planning process in 1993, with the National Vaccine Program Office (NVPO) as the lead agency. After the 1997 Hong Kong outbreak, to which the CDC was a major responder, Shalala ordered NVPO to prepare technical content for a federal response plan; HHS also established a liaison committee on pandemic influenza with the Department of Defense, the Federal Emergency Management Agency (FEMA), and the Red Cross. Much of this, however, was simply bureaucratic rewiring that provided little incentive for vaccine development or re-investment in local public-health agencies.

In October 2000, the GAO scolded HHS for making so little progress in the development of an avian flu vaccine. It warned that the United States might only have a month (or less) of warning before a pandemic became widespread, and it accused HHS of failing to develop contingency plans to ensure expanded vaccine manufacturing capacity. It also pointed to a major contradiction in business-as-usual reliance on the private sector: "Because no market exists for vaccine after [flu season], manufacturers switch their capacity to other uses between about mid-August and December." At minimum, HHS needed to find some way to keep production lines running full-time, all year long, as well as to diversify the number of companies committed to vaccine production. In addition, the GAO slammed HHS for dithering over whether or not to stockpile antivirals, even as top influenza experts were begging the government to procure as much oseltamivir (Tamiflu)—the "miracle" neuraminidase inhibitor—as possible. Finally, the audit faulted Shalala's department for poor coordination of the respective roles of the federal government, state agencies, and private manufacturers. Almost eight years of "process," the GAO report implied, had failed to achieve a "plan" in any substantive or meaningful sense.[241]

Meanwhile, the Republican leadership in Congress, after driving a silver stake through Clinton's health insurance reform, slashed at programs that even faintly smacked of social entitlement. Federal funding for state immunization programs (which Clinton had dramatically increased) was a principal target, with aid cut in some cases by more than 50 percent. As a 2000 study by the National Institutes of Health (NIH) emphasized, influenza vaccination already lagged far behind its potential to prevent disease and death. NIH pointed to glaring racial and income disparities in flu vaccine coverage, attributing the low vaccination rates among blacks (22 percent), Latinos (19 percent), and the uninsured (14 percent) to federal cutbacks as well as the increased dependence of Americans upon tightwad HMOs for their medical care.[242] Another study by researchers at the University of Rochester found that only 39 percent of black people over age sixty-five received influenza vaccinations as compared with 71 percent of white seniors.[243] There was—and is—still a color line in prevention of flu mortality.

As the GAO constantly reminded Congress, the U.S. hospital system could no longer deal with pandemics or mass casualties of any kind. The restructuring of health care around HMOs, with the attendant closure of hundreds of hospitals across the United States, had left many big cities without the capacity to deal with abnormal spikes in patient loads; the HMO ideal was to ruthlessly reduce the number of unused, and thus unprofitable, hospital beds to zero: an example of "just-in-time" management gone berserk. Public hospitals, meanwhile, were caught between their chronic budgetary problems and soaring demand by the more than 40 million poor and uninsured Americans. A 2003 survey by the American College of Emergency Physicians found that 90 percent of the country's 4,000 emergency departments were seriously understaffed and overcrowded, with little surge capacity.[244]

Influenza experts point to the ominous experience of Los Angeles during the H3N2/Sidney epidemic in the winter of 1997/98 as a precursor to things to come. Having lost 17 percent of their beds since 1990, Los Angeles County hospitals were overwhelmed by an unexpected influx of flu patients, hardly reassuring evidence of the system's capacity to deal with a real pandemic crisis.[245] After the 2002 election the Institute of Medicine looked back glumly at the Bush senior and Clinton epochs. It found that many of its past recommendations had never been implemented and that the public-health system "that was in disarray in 1988 remains in disarray today."[246]

This "disarray," including all the flaws in HHS's influenza program (particularly the lack of an antiviral stockpile and adequate vaccine manufacturing capacity), was inherited by Tommy Thompson, the former governor of Wisconsin, described as a "pragmatic conservative" by his friend Ted Kennedy. The Clinton administration's handling of public-health issues had certainly been disappointing, but the new Bush administration was frightening to everyone who had been fighting to prevent the total meltdown of urban public health. Then, in September 2001, a new dispensation suddenly arrived in the form of poisoned letters contaminated with "weaponized" anthrax. DNA sequencing would later reveal that the anthrax strain used in the attacks almost certainly originated from the Army's own laboratory at Fort Detrick, Maryland, yet this probable "inside job" became the principal justification for national hysteria about the threat of "bioterrorism" supposedly posed by Iraq, al-Qaeda, and other alien enemies of the United States.[247]

With shockingly little debate and without any real evidence that such a threat even existed, most public-health advocacy groups, as well as such leading Democrats as John Edwards and Ted Kennedy, became ardent shareholders in the bioterrorism myth. Even the liberal Trust for America's Health glibly talked of an "Age of Bioterrorism" as if malevolent hands were already opening little vials of botulism and Ebola on Main Street. In fact, the irresistible attraction of the so-called "health/security nexus" was the billions that the White House was proposing to spend on Project BioShield, Bush's "major research and production effort to guard our people against bioterrorism." Many well-meaning people undoubtedly reasoned that, however farfetched the excuse, the Republicans were finally throwing money in a worthwhile direction and that some of the windfall would surely find its way to real needs after decades of neglect. Because the defensive preparations against bioterrorism borrowed heavily from pandemic planning, there was hope that influenza (previously shortchanged in the design of the National Pharmaceutical Stockpile in 1999) would be accorded its proper rank as a "most wanted" bioterrorist.

Certainly the leading influenza researchers, from 2001 onwards, were doing their utmost to alert medical colleagues worldwide to the urgent threat of avian flu, as well as outlining the immediate steps that the Bush administration and other governments needed to take. As befitted his position as "pope" of influenza researchers, Robert Webster tirelessly preached the same sermon: "If a pandemic happened today, hospital facilities would be overwhelmed and understaffed because many medical personnel would be afflicted with the disease [the lesson of SARS]. Vaccine production would be slow because many drug-company employees would also be victims. Critical community services would be immobilized. Reserves of existing vaccines, M2 inhibitors, and NA inhibitors would be quickly depleted, leaving most people vulnerable to infection."[248]

Webster stressed the particular urgency of increasing production of the neuraminidase (NA) inhibitor oseltamivir (Tamiflu).* Because a vaccine was unlikely to be available in the early stages of a pandemic, Webster urged that "NA inhibitors [e.g. oseltamivir] should be stockpiled now, in huge quantities." Because this strategic antiviral was "in woefully short supply"—made by Roche at a single factory in Switzerland—Webster and his colleagues underlined the need for resolute government action. "The cost of making the drugs, as opposed to the price the pharmaceutical companies charge consumers, would not be exorbitant. Such expenditure by governments would be a very worthwhile investment in the defence against this debilitating and often deadly virus." Failure to act would mean intense

* The other neuraminidase inhibitor, zanamivir (Relenza), is equally effective, but it is an inhaled drug in short supply, not as attractive a candidate for stockpiling as the much easier-to-use Tamiflu.

competition over the small inventory of life-saving Tamiflu. "Who should get these drugs? Health-care workers and those in essential services, obviously, but who would identify these? There would not be nearly enough for those who needed them in the developed world, let alone the rest of the world's population."[249]

Webster was not calling for a new Manhattan Project, just prudent action to ensure an adequate antiviral stockpile. But for almost three years he and other influenza experts were ignored, as were those who argued more generally that "the best way to manage bioterrorism is to improve the management of existing public health threats."[250] The Bush administration instead fast-tracked vaccination programs for smallpox and anthrax, based on fanciful scenarios that might have embarrassed Tom Clancy. In reality, Project BioShield was designed to build support for the invasion of Iraq by sowing the baseless fear that Saddam Hussein might use bioweapons against the United States.* In any event, Washington spent $1 billion expanding a smallpox vaccine stockpile that some experts claim was already quite sufficient. Hundreds of thousands of GIs were forced to undergo the vaccinations, but frontline health workers—the second tier of the smallpox campaign—largely boycotted the administration's attempts to cajole "voluntary" participation.

In spite of this fiasco and millions of doses of unused vaccine, the administration pressed ahead with the development of second-generation smallpox and anthrax vaccines, as well as vaccines for such exotic plagues as Ebola fever; it continued to

---

* By militarizing the biotechnology sector, BioShield also obviously aims to woo young science entrepreneurs and their startup firms to the Republican Party.

reject the "all hazards" strategy recommended by most public-health experts in favor of a so-called "siloed approach" that focused on a shortlist of possible bioweapons. In testimony before the House of Representatives, Tommy Thompson explained that while "private investment should drive the development of most medical products," only the government was in a position to develop those products that "everyone hopes . . . will never be needed" as a protection against "rare yet deadly threats." The government, in other words, was willing to spend lots of money on biological threats that were unlikely or far-fetched, but not on antivirals or new antibiotics for the diseases that were actually most menacing. As Project BioShield morphed into the biggest show in town (growing from $3 billion in fiscal 2002 to more than $5 billion in fiscal 2004), Thompson's wayward logic soon had perverse impacts that confounded the hopes of the biodefense boom's early enthusiasts.[251]

For example, instead of spurring a welcome trickle-down of money for research on big killers like influenza, malaria, and tuberculosis, BioShield stole top laboratory talent away from major disease research. With the National Institutes of Health's research budget barely keeping pace with inflation (after its banquet days under Clinton), there was an irresistible tropism of researchers and research projects toward biodefense windfalls. Reporting on this new "brain drain," writer Merrill Goozner cited the case of a leading UCLA lab that phased out its "basic science research on TB in favor of studying tularemia [rabbit fever]"—a disease that "has zero public-health importance"—because the latter infection was "on the government's A-list of potential bioterrorism agents" and tuberculosis was not.[252] (After workers at a different lab accidentally infected themselves with tularemia, some scientists expressed concern to the *New York Times* that "leaky" biodefense research "may pose a menace to public health comparable to the still uncertain threat from bioterrorism.")[253]

To many infectious disease experts, Project BioShield was Bush's and Thompson's version of *Through the Looking Glass*, with priorities established in inverse relationship to actual probabilities of attack or outbreak. "It's too bad that Saddam Hussein's not behind influenza," complained Dr. Paul Offitt, a dissident member of the government's advisory panel on vaccination. "We'd be doing a better job."[254] Indeed, HHS's zeal to combat hypothetical bioterrorism contrasted with its incredible negligence in exercising oversight over the nation's "fragile" influenza vaccine supply. As the GAO had warned Donna Shalala, vaccine availability in a pandemic would depend upon the stability and surge capacity of existing production lines. But as shocked Americans discovered in the winter of 2003–4 and again in early fall 2004, the entire vaccine manufacturing system had decayed almost to the point of collapse. While Bush and Thompson were trying to bribe the pharmaceutical industry to join Project BioShield, the same industry was abdicating its elementary responsibility to maintain a lifeline of new vaccines and antibiotics.

"Big Pharma," as recent exposés have emphasized, is the most profitable industry in the United States, and it maintains the most powerful lobby on Capitol Hill. (According to Harvard Medical School's Marcia Angell, the ten big drug companies included in the *Fortune* 500 in 2002 earned more in profit than all the other 490 corporations combined.)[255] Thanks to the tolerance of a Congress awash in its campaign contributions, the

drug industry mines gold from outrageous prescription prices
for drugs that manage chronic illness (diabetes, high blood pressure, asthma, and so on), as well as the sale of such lifestyle en-
hancers as Viagra.

Products that actually cure or prevent disease, like vaccines
and antibiotics, are less profitable, so infectious disease has largely
become an orphan market. As industry analysts point out, worldwide sales for *all* vaccines produce less revenue than Pfizer's income from a single anticholesterol medication.[256] Despite the
90,000 Americans who die every year from hospital infections,
the drug corporations also scorn spending money on the development of new antibiotics. Indeed, as *Nature* writer Martin
Leeb points out, "from a marketing standpoint, antibiotics are
the worst sort of pharmaceutical because they cure the disease."[257] The giants prefer to invest in marketing rather than research, in rebranded old products rather than new ones, and in
treatment rather than prevention, in fact, they currently spend
27 percent of their revenue on marketing and only 11 percent
on research. (Not surprisingly, "all the CEOs of major pharmaceutical companies [are] from marketing and sales; they are not
scientists.")[258] "Preventing a flu epidemic that could kill thousands," wrote Donald Barlett and James Steele in *Time* magazine, "is not nearly as profitable as making pills for something
like erectile dysfunction."[259]

11

Structural Contradictions

One of the most difficult things to explain to the public after a pandemic would be why we weren't prepared, because there have been enough warnings.[260]

Klaus Stohr, WHO

Influenza vaccines are especially disliked by drug companies because they are tricky to produce, become obsolete after one season, and are subject to large fluctuations in demand. Moreover, the basic production process has changed little since the days of Francis and Salk a half century ago, and the industry has failed to invest in the faster and safer cell-culture technology that would eliminate the risk of contamination inherent in using fertile chicken eggs.[261] Vaccine manufacturing in general is widely regarded as a broken-down old railroad to be off-loaded at the first opportunity rather than repaired and modernized. Big Pharma, by and large, has spurned the little biotech startups in San Diego, Austin, and Boston that have been searching for capital to develop exciting new recombinant and genetically engineered vaccines. In terms of vaccine development in general, the United States measures poorly even against tiny Cuba which, thanks to the priority given to infectious and "poor people's" diseases, has become a world leader in creating state-of-the-art vaccines for meningitis B, *Haemophilus influenzae*, and other important infections ignored by giant drug companies in the United States.[262]

Meanwhile, aging and poorly maintained vaccine production facilities have been plagued by poor quality control and indifferent management. In September 2000, for example, 12 percent of the influenza vaccine supply was lost when the FDA shut down Parkdale Pharmaceuticals' contaminated facility, which never reopened; deliveries from Wyeth-Ayerst, which produced one-third of the national supply, were also delayed because of quality problems (the company abandoned vaccine production two years later after a mild flu season left millions of doses unsold).[263] By the winter of 2003–4—with the Institute of Medicine sternly warning Washington that the country was still "poorly prepared" for a flu pandemic—only two corporations were still making influenza vaccine for the U.S. market: French-owned Aventis-Pasteur with a manufacturing complex in Swiftwater, Pennsylvania, and Bay Area-based Chiron, with a recently acquired plant near Liverpool.[264]

This was an extraordinary contrast to the situation in 1976, when *thirty-seven* companies in the United States produced flu vaccine, or for that matter, to current policy in the UK, where the government retains contracts with six major suppliers.[265] Although the GAO had warned HHS in May 2001 about the "fragility of the vaccine supply," the Department "didn't display any comprehension of what the problem was and what should be done about it."[266] Even as it hyped the importance of "biosecurity," the Bush administration in essence mortgaged the lives of tens of thousands of senior citizens, for whom annual influenza is a life-threatening illness, by relying on vaccine production in just two plants—and one of them, it would turn out, had an alarming record of poor quality control.

The 2003–4 flu season brought another vaccine disaster: a virulent strain of annual influenza (H3N2 Fujian), which was not included in the vaccine mixture, proved more dangerous than expected to small children, and the old-fashioned egg-based production system precluded any last-minute reformulation of the vaccine. Even with a component missing, vaccine demand rose steeply; however, the two manufacturers, wary of being stuck with an excess supply as they had been the previous year, had manufactured too little, and some localities had to resort to rationing. While HHS had foreseen the likely shortfall, they had failed to exert enough pressure on the manufacturers to increase production.

As the media headlined stories about children in Texas and Colorado dying from the Fujian strain, the CDC was nervously monitoring the new, extraordinarily widespread outbreak of H5N1 in Asia. Secretary Thompson finally acknowledged—although with less urgency than previous announcements about anthrax and smallpox—that a flu pandemic was an imminent danger, and the administration promised to accelerate vaccine development. Despite widespread criticism of their conduct during the previous flu season, Thompson decided to again make Aventis-Pasteur and Chiron the twin pillars of the U.S. vaccine program. In May both corporations received contracts from the National Institute of Allergy and Infectious Diseases to produce experimental lots of an H5N1 vaccine using a seed strain from Robert Webster's laboratory at St. Jude; in mid-August, Chiron was also awarded the contract to develop a vaccine against the H9N2 subtype.

In retrospect, it is hard to fathom Thompson's confidence in Chiron. Under a succession of previous owners, its Liverpool plant had developed a notorious reputation for contamination. "It is an antiquated facility and poorly managed" was the opinion of one business analyst.[267] British authorities had once recalled contaminated polio vaccines made in the plant, while the FDA had admonished a previous owner about impurities in its flu vaccine. In the summer of 2003 FDA inspectors discovered significant risk of bacterial contamination in twenty different production activities, especially in the sterilization processes; because the plant was responsible for manufacturing almost half of the U.S. vaccine supply, the inspection team recommended compulsory steps to mitigate the danger. Their superiors, however, insisted upon voluntary, rather than mandatory, compliance. The agency then curiously delayed for nine months before forwarding Chiron its full inspection report, and, instead of sending inspectors back to monitor Chiron's progress, FDA officials consulted with the company by telephone or email. Lester Crawford, the acting head of the FDA, later assured a skeptical congressional committee that since the 2003–4 vaccine was acceptable, the FDA considered Chiron's Liverpool problems resolved. ("They had in fact completed what we wanted them to do.")[268]

The FDA's timidity and Crawford's nonchalance angered U.S. Representative Henry Waxman of California and other members of the House Committee on Government Reform, but they also knew that the agency's policy of sleeping with the enemy, or rather, "working with the pharmaceutical industry as a trusted partner," had been promoted by the Clinton administration—supposedly in order to speed production and approval of "breakthrough drugs." Critics of Big Pharma, on the other hand, saw the FDA's "partnership" with Chiron as classic evidence that another regulatory agency had been captured by the industry it was supposed to regulate.

In July 2004 Chiron found *Serratia marcescens*—a bacteria that can cause deadly septic shock—in several batches of vaccine. Instead of immediately alerting the FDA, the company instead issued a press release "boasting that it already had shipped 1 million doses of Fluviron vaccine to the U.S. market and planned to ship 52 million more doses." Chiron waited more than a month, until 26 August, to notify the FDA of contamination. Once again, Crawford trusted the corporation to rectify the problem. At the end of September, Chiron CEO Howard Pien personally reassured the Senate Committee on Aging that quality control had been restored to the Liverpool plant, which would soon ship 48 million doses of vaccine to the United States; instead, a week later, vigilant British inspectors shut the plant down and revoked Chiron's license to sell flu vaccine.[269] Although the corporation claimed that a portion of the vaccine was uncontaminated, FDA investigators determined that the entire stock was spoiled.

As a result, the United States lost half of its seasonal vaccine and was forced to ration the rest. Although the CDC and local health officials worked miracles in shifting vaccine to areas of greatest need, the crazy quiltwork of the U.S. vaccine distribution system—with literally thousands of independent government and private agents involved—gave a disturbing foretaste of the chaos that a pandemic would create. The Chiron disaster easily risked killing as many Americans through lack of vaccination as the 9/11 attacks, but Thompson, Crawford, and their underlings continued to breezily disclaim any responsibility for errors of oversight. Amazingly they also let Chiron keep its contracts for manufacturing avian flu vaccines.

As public anger grew over the fiasco, which was soon followed by shocking exposes of the FDA's failure to monitor drug safety in a variety of cases, even the mainstream media was forced to acknowledge structural contradictions in the system. Thus, the *New York Times*, in a moment of almost Marxist revelation, identified the underlying problem as the "chronic mismatch of public health needs and private control of the production of vaccines and drugs."[270] (In August, the HHS's draft National Pandemic Influenza Preparedness Plan had made a similar point in more cautious language, noting that the United States's "primarily private vaccine purchase and delivery system may not be optimal in a pandemic.")[271]

The vaccine crisis also prompted closer scrutiny of other major components of the pandemic plan which in its snail's pace evolution since 1993 had finally arrived at the final comment and discussion phase in fall 2004. The *New York Times*—the only major newspaper that seemed to take avian flu seriously—published an editorial on 12 October chastising HHS for proposing to add only 2 million courses of oseltamivir (Tamiflu) to the Strategic National Stockpile. The editors pointed out that while Japan had purchased enough Tamiflu for 20 percent of its population, and Australia for 5 percent, the Bush administration's order would cover less than 1 percent of Americans. "Ten times that amount," said the *Times*, "would seem more reasonable. The drug favored in this country is made by a single manufacturer whose capacity is limited, but a contract for massive quantities would presumably energize the industry to ramp up production."[272]

In fact, there was gridlock in Switzerland, where Roche had failed to expand capacity to keep pace with its overflowing order book. The manufacturer recommended that governments stockpile enough Tamiflu to cover one-quarter of their populations, the estimated infection rate of an influenza pandemic; this rule of thumb would mandate 1.6 billion courses globally, with 74 million for the United States. Roche's recommendations might have been self-serving, but they were not far-fetched: Dr. Julie Gerberding, the head of the CDC, told the *New York Times* that she would like to see a U.S. stockpile closer to 100 million courses than 1 million. But in fall 2004 Roche, although it was trying to add a new production line, was only producing 8 million courses per year. "Some public health experts," the *Times* reported, "are strongly critical of Roche for not increasing production of Tamiflu sooner, saying that the company should have expanded production this year, when avian influenza started becoming a problem across much of Asia."[273]

The obvious solution to both the Tamiflu shortage and the vaccine fiasco is for the federal government itself to undertake the nonprofit development and manufacture of lifeline medications. But in a political system where almost everyone dances to the tune of the drug industry's political contributions, the "liberal" alternative to the Bush administration's negligence was the proposal, supported by presidential candidate John Kerry and other Democrats, to raise market demand with larger government purchases. Meanwhile, for the foreseeable future Americans would be trapped in precisely the dilemma that Robert Webster had warned about: How should the scarce supply of Tamiflu, the only antiviral known to be effective against avian influenza, be rationed? Americans would be faced with a veritable "Sophie's choice": who would come first, frontline health workers or their most vulnerable patients? Elderly people or babies? Young mothers or policemen? Or perhaps the imperial legions should be protected first? In late September the Pentagon circulated its own pandemic planning guidelines which emphasized that the Tamiflu "supply is extremely limited world wide, and its use will be prioritized." The military's "top priority for use of vaccine or antiviral medications is in forward deployed operational forces. . . . We are currently working with HHS on agreements to share in the HHS/CDC Strategic National Stockpile (SNS)."[274] Soldiers first, children last?

Such questions deeply trouble the medical community. At a 2002 meeting of public-health officials from forty-six different states, participants were hopelessly divided when they tried to choose which of five goals (reduce deaths, reduce disease, limit impact, ensure essential services, or "equitable distribution") should be paramount in allocation of scarce antivirals.[275] More recently, in August 2004, the American College of Physicians and the American Society of Internal Medicine jointly expressed concerns about the CDC's proposal to ration any future avian flu vaccine among vulnerable groups, stating a "strong consensus among our group that limiting vaccine to specific target groups suggested by CDC may be less than optimal." In October Dr. Andrew Parvia, the chair of the Infectious Diseases Society of America's pandemic influenza taskforce, reported similar concerns to the society's annual conference. He emphasized the need for clear, consistent guidelines for "triage," and he proposed that pneumococcal vaccines that reduce the likelihood of secondary infections be added to the pandemic stockpile. He also criticized the Bush administration's miserly budget for pandemic influenza: Pavia stated that the proposed $100 million "seriously underestimates the amount of funds realistically needed to effectively respond to the next pandemic."[276]

Meanwhile, grim audits of the nation's real biosecurity situation were piling up at Tommy Thompson's doorstep. Michael Osterholm, the director of the University of Minnesota's Center for Infectious Disease Research and Policy, garnered much press attention with a warning that the H5N1 vaccine that the National Institutes of Health had been developing with Aventis-Pasteur had "poor immunogenicity" (ability to trigger an immune response). Osterholm warned: "The earlier versions of this vaccine are not protective against the current [H5N1] strains." He doubted that the government's slow-motion vaccine program would provide a safety net in advance of a pandemic. "In the early stages of a pandemic I don't believe we will have a pandemic influenza vaccine of any substantive nature."[277] (This echoed the offical pandemic plan's own pessimistic prediction that in the beginning of an outbreak "there will likely be no or very limited amounts of vaccine available. This period could last for up to six months.")[278] Keiji Fukuda, the CDC's top flu epidemiologist, direly predicted that at the beginning of a pandemic "there would be panic" and that hospitals would be unable to find room for all the acute cases.[279]

Similarly, in the aftermath of the vaccine fiasco, both the *Washington Post* and the nonprofit Trust for America's Health published devastating balance-sheets revealing Project BioShield's failure to enhance the country's biological security. The *Post* reporters, who interviewed former administration officials, found that the "great majority of U.S. hospitals and state and local public health agencies would be completely overwhelmed trying to carry out mass vaccinations." And indeed, during a May 2003 mock casualty exercise to test Chicago's capacity to cope with a bioterror attack or a pandemic, the emergency infrastructure collapsed. Richard A. Falkenrath, a former chief advisor on homeland security, told the *Post* that "the government's reliance on state and local health agencies to speedily distribute vaccines and drugs is the 'Achilles heel' of U.S. biodefenses." In obvious understatement, the *Post* characterized as "vast" the task of "redirecting cash-starved hospitals and local health agencies into the unfamiliar field of mass casualty response."[280]

The Trust for America's Health was equally pessimistic. One-third of states had cut back their public-health budgets in 2003–4, and a majority were woefully unprepared to undertake high biosecurity lab work, to distribute vaccines, or to track outbreaks. Although "most public health officials call the emergence of a new lethal strain of the flu 'an inevitability,'" only thirteen states had pandemic plans that met federal guidelines, while twenty states had failed to generate any plan. Earlier in February 2004, the Trust had warned that "pandemic flu could be much more demanding on state and local health resources and much more damaging to the general population than a bioterrorism attack." It predicted that a pandemic would "cripple the resources of a U.S. public health system already stretched too thin."[281]

In short, as *Nature* pointed out, "Three years of heightened concern about bioterrorism have done nothing to address the fundamental weakness of the U.S. public health system."[282] Except for those lucky few—mainly doctors and soldiers—who might receive prophylactic treatment with Tamiflu, the Bush administration had left most Americans as vulnerable to the onslaught of a new flu pandemic as their grandparents or great-grandparents had been in 1918. Pandemic planners admitted that the bulk of the public, initially at least, would simply have to cower in their homes. In a presidential election season dominated by "national security," pandemic vulnerability should have been a decisive wedge issue; however, the Kerry campaign scolded Bush for the vaccine debacle and promised to stabilize future production with government purchases of unused stocks, but otherwise offered few substantive ideas for repairing America's collapsing public–health infrastructure.[283] Kerry, in fact, let Bush off the hook, never once mentioning the avian influenza threat in any of the three presidential debates.

The only presidential candidate to pay attention to the monster at the door was Ralph Nader, the candidate whose presence in the campaign was so reviled by "progressive" born-again Democrats. In February 2004 Nader contrasted the administration's obsession with Iraq's nonexistent "weapons of mass destruction" with its failure to energetically address avian flu in Asia. "The chain of infections from domesticated Chinese ducks to pigs to humans," he forewarned in colorful prose, "can explode into a world war of mutant viruses taking millions of casualties before vaccines can be developed and deployed." Six months later he wrote a public letter to Bush impeaching the administration's failure to act upon the warnings of top researchers and medical organizations. "Such notice apparently is not enough to move your Presidency to action. These mutating viruses are not like human villains. You need to recognize that their indiscriminate destruction of innocent civilians, however, can be considered a form of viral terrorism."[284] In the WHO's "worst-case" scenario, 2 million of these "innocent civilians" threatened with death are Americans, most of the remaining 98 million, however, live in the poor cities of the Third World.

12

The *Titanic* Paradigm

*Access to medicines has become the test above
all others by which the rich world will be judged
in its dealings with the poor.*[285]

Richard Horton

Scientific agreement about the imminent danger of an avian flu
pandemic is almost as broad and all-encompassing as the consensus that humans are largely responsible for global warming.
All the summit organizations responsible for world health, including the WHO and the CDC, have warned that the coming
viral hurricane might be even more deadly than the 1918 pandemic. The major dissenter to this view is Amherst biologist
Paul Ewald, a controversial advocate of "evolutionary medicine." In his view, the leading influenza experts have failed to
grasp elementary principles of viral evolution, especially "the
selective processes that favor increased or decreased virulence of
virus strains." The 1918 pandemic, in his view, was a unique historical event whose catastrophic outcome depended upon the
evolution of influenza virulence in the extraordinary conditions
of the Western Front. "Both theory and the evidence," he
claims, "implicate the Western Front as the source of the epidemic." Ewald doubts that environmental conditions so favorable

to the emergence of hypervirulence in influenza A will ever reappear. "We will fail to see," he predicts, "a recurrence of a pandemic influenza with the kind of lethality that characterized the 1918 pandemic."[286]

Some scholars, of course, would dispute that the virulent second wave of the 1918 virus originated in France at all: Kansas, in fact, seems a better bet. Ewald also skirts over the geography of the great pandemic, whose deadly epicenter was India, not the Western Front; nor does he engage theories about how malnutrition and malaria amplified influenza mortality. Still, Ewald may be correct that crowded Army training camps, hospitals, and ships, as well as the trenches themselves, were the bellows that turned outbreak into conflagration. The 1918 pandemic dramatically grew in virulence between its initial spring outbreak and the deadly second wave in the early fall, so the key variables must have been crowded, often unsanitary conditions with large concentrations of sick victims able to transmit an evolving virus quickly to distant locations. Ewald calls such an environment a "disease factory."[287] He might also have called it a slum.

The Western Front of the world's first industrialized war recapitulated much of the disease ecology of the classic Victorian slum—the *locus classicus* of most discourse about infectious disease. In the nineteenth century, the great slums of Europe, America, and Asia had a total population of perhaps 25 million; today, according to UN-Habitat, there are 1 billion slum-dwellers: a number expected to double by 2020. Is there any reason to assume that today's *bustees, colonias,* and shantytowns are any less efficient "disease factories" than Victorian slums or crowded 1918 army camps? If, according to Ewald, the *sine qua non* of a deadly airborne pandemic is "host density" in poor sanitary conditions, then—as Table 12.1 shows—today's megaslums are just as fetid and overcrowded as any of their notorious Victorian predecessors. With population densities as high as 200,000 residents per square kilometer, they offer perfect environments for the evolution of flu virulence. By such criteria, pandemic influenza and other deadly infections have a brilliant future.

While the combustible role of Asia's thousands of slums in the development of a future pandemic has been oddly neglected in the research literature, the great concentrations of urban poverty in Dhaka, Kolkata, Mumbai, and Karachi are presumably like so many lakes of gasoline waiting for the spark of H5N1. Moreover, the contemporary megaslum may be a crucial link in a new global disease ecology. In 1976 the historian William McNeill proposed that there had been three "historic transitions" in the co-evolution of humans and microbes: the Neolithic (agro-urban) revolution; the creation of an Eurasian Ecumene in classical times; and the rise of the modern world system in the sixteenth century. Each transition was a stage in the biological "reunification" of the human race as well as a corresponding exchange of microbial parasites. Some epidemiologists now argue that neoliberal globalization represents a fourth transition or "reshaping of relations between humans and microbes."[288] Clearly, the crucial environmental conditions favoring the rise of a new pandemic flu offer a partial model of this larger transitional dynamic.

To recapitulate from earlier chapters, the two global changes that have most favored the accelerated cross-species evolution of novel influenza subtypes and their global transmission have been

Table 12.1.
Urban Density (1000s per km^2)

(Slums in Italics)

Dharavi (Mumbai—densest streets)	571.0
Delhi (densest slum)	300.0
Kibera (Nairobi)	200.0
Cite-Soleil (Port-au-Prince)	180.0
Lower East Side (1910)	145.0
City of Dead (Cairo)	116.0
Les Halles (Paris, 1850s)	100.0
Imbaba (Cairo)	84.0
Dhaka (old town)	80.0
Five Points (New York, 1850)	77.0
Nairobi slums (average)	63.0
Orangi (Karachi)	50.0
Manhattan (1910)	32.0
Cairo (greater) & Caracas *barrios*	25.0
Mumbai & Lagos	20.0
Colonias populares (Mex. City)	19.0
Shanghai	16.4
Manhattan & central Tokyo	13.4
Mexico City	11.7
World urban average	**6.6**
London	4.5
Los Angeles	2.4

the Livestock Revolution of the 1980–90s (part of the larger world conquest of agriculture by large-scale agro-capitalism) and the industrial revolution in South China (the historical crucible of human influenzas) which has exponentially increased the region's commercial and human intercourse with the rest of the world. The emergence of Third World "supercities" and their slums, then, would constitute a third global condition tantamount to Ewald's Western Front as a human medium for potential pandemic spread and virulence evolution.

(One of Ewald's signal theoretical contributions to the study of pandemics, by the way, has been to show that pathogens do not always become less virulent and more well-behaved over time, as some textbooks still claim. Offered the unprecedented menu of huge slum populations, a new pandemic influenza might not be as easily tamed as some of its ancestors. As Ewald explains, "If predator-like variants of a pathogen population out-produce and out-transmit benign pathogens, then peaceful coexistence and long-term stability may be precluded much as it is often precluded in predator-prey systems.")[289]

But there is also a fourth, negative element that closes the ominous circle of influenza ecology: the absence of an international public health system corresponding to the scale and impact of economic globalization. Such a system, as Laurie Garrett emphasizes in her much-praised book, *Betrayal of Trust: The Collapse of Global Public Health*, "would have to embrace not just the essential elements of disease prevention and surveillance that were present in wealthy pockets of the planet during the twentieth century, but also new strategies and tactics capable of addressing global challenges." Nothing like this, of course, now exists, and Garrett paints a dark, almost despairing portrait of how the worldwide HMO revolution (which, in addition its effect into the United States, has also had a surprisingly broad impact on developing countries) has promoted cost-containment at the expense of saving lives. The WHO, "once the conscience of global health," Garrett adds "lost its way in the 1990s. Demoralized, rife with rumors of corruption, and lacking in leadership, the WHO floundered."[290]

Richard Horton, the editor of *The Lancet*, the premier British medical journal, offers an equally bleak view of world public health. "UNICEF and WHO have largely abandoned the world's children to die in poverty. For example, spending on immunization by UNICEF totaled $180 million in 1990. By 1998, the figure had fallen to around $50 million." Some 11 million children under the age of five die each year, and "99 per cent of these deaths occur in setting of acute poverty." Horton accuses the WHO, even under the supposedly enlightened tenure of Director-General Gro Harlem Brundtland, both of being subservient to corporate elites and "of censorship when criticism was made of the pharmaceutical industry." He also damns the Bush administration's sordid crusade to defend Big Pharma's monopoly over drugs treating chronic conditions. "Once again," he wrote after a 2002 U.S. veto of Third World efforts to obtain cheaper generic pharmaceuticals, "access to vital drugs to treat health emergencies among those living in poverty will be restricted solely to protect profit. And WHO has nothing to say on this issue." Many of the most effective artemisinin-based antimalarial drugs, for example, are priced out of reach of the poor people whose infants and small children die in such shocking numbers every year in sub-Saharan Africa.[291]

Many Third World governments, meanwhile, are disinclined

to spend much on public health when the alternative is feeding their generals' bottomless appetites for new weapons. Delhi, for instance, spends 16 percent of its budget on defense, but only 2 percent ($4 per capita per annum) on health.[292] Other poor countries are too shackled by structural adjustment and debt to have any choice. "Kenya," Alex de Waal complains, "finds itself unable to offer jobs to several thousand unemployed nurses because of a cap on public-sector employment, while Zambia is in the extraordinary position of being required to lay off health-sector employees, even while many districts have no health professionals at all."[293] In sub-Saharan Africa, where 100,000 trained medical workers were lost during the 1990s to AIDS or emigration, it is estimated that the region desperately needs at least 1 million more personnel, especially nurses and assistants, to ensure even the most rudimentary public-health coverage to the entire population.[294]

In the face of the peril of avian influenza, as with HIV/AIDS earlier, world public health resources are organized rather like the lifeboats were on the Titanic: many of the first-class passengers and even some of the crew will drown because of the company's skinflint lack of foresight; the poor Paddies in steerage, however, do not even have a single lifeboat between them, and thus, they are all doomed to swim in the icy waters. In September 2004, with H5N1 resuming its murderous course in Vietnam, local authorities and the WHO were desperate to vaccinate exposed populations to prevent a possible reassortment of avian and human influenzas. But as WHO influenza chief Klaus Stohr bitterly complained to the *New Scientist,* "There is no excess. There is no vaccine available for Vietnam." Thailand, although much wealthier than Vietnam, faced the same problem. "We do not have sufficient vaccine to prevent co-circulation," complained Prasert Thongcharoen, a prominent representative to the WHO. What little surplus was available in Europe and Canada had been bought up by New York City and other local U.S. health authorities in the wake of the Chiron fiasco.[295]

Only twelve drug companies make influenza vaccines, and fully 95 percent of their output (about 260 million doses) is consumed in the world's wealthiest countries. Current production is limited by the supply of fertile eggs, and even a switch to cell culture—as all experts advocate—would face the problem that "there are surprisingly few suitable accredited cell lines and cell banks available, and many of those are the property of pharmaceutical companies."[296] Despite the WHO's urgent Geneva summit in October to lobby governments to finance (and drug companies to produce) a so-called "world vaccine," little progress has been made. "Of the world's major flu vaccine manufacturers," *Science* reported during the summit, "so far only two are willing to tackle the financial, regulatory and patent issues involved in making a new pandemic vaccine, mainly for the U.S. market."[297] Previous test vaccines, as we have seen, failed to keep pace with the evolving virulence of H5N1, and even if current clinical trials are successful, Washington has ordered only 2 million doses from Aventis-Pasteur. With the exception of Canada (which has contracted with a Quebec-based firm to gear up production for 6 million doses per month), most wealthy countries are buying just a few "lifeboats" now in the dubious belief that they will have time to order more when the crisis arrives. (A recent Johns Hopkins study shows that, unlike the 1968 pandemic, which took a year to circle the world, air travel would now spread a pandemic much faster than pharmaceutical factories could be geared up to produce vaccine.)[298]

With so little investment in expanded manufacturing capacity, the WHO came up with a desperate scheme to stretch the vaccine supply by adding a cheap adjuvant like alum. (Unfortunately, some researchers believe that even with adjuvants, two doses may be needed to make an H5N1 vaccine effective, a possibility that would double the problem.)[299] Stohr urged EU leaders to take the initiative in testing a low-dose pandemic H5N1 vaccine containing an adjuvant. While he argued that this was the only possible way to ensure that some vaccine would be available to the Third World, Europe could not find the money. "The EU," Stohr caustically observed, "has not the flexibility or the political will."[300] *Nature* echoed Stohr in rebuking the EU for failing to support pandemic planning and accelerated vaccine development.[301]

Without vaccines, as we have seen, there will be a mad global scramble over Tamiflu: according to *Science* "the world's only initial defense against a pandemic that could kill millions."[302] Back in 1999, René Snacken, the chair of the European Scientific Working Group on Influenza, warned that "waiting until a pandemic strikes to determine access to prophylactic materials inevitably contributes to inequities in supply for countries to produce antiviral agents or vaccines or lacking resources to competitively purchase supplies at a time of scarcity."[303] The WHO, of course, has stressed the "need for international solidarity"; arguing that the only way to contain an initial pandemic outbreak will be to douse it with powerful antivirals. It has urged the pooling of Tamiflu for use in Southeast

Asia. "But whether countries will voluntarily ship their own precious stockpiles overseas to fight a faraway plague remains to be seen."[304] Even if some antivirals are made available, there is little guarantee they will actually reach people in the hot spots. In 2004, for example, all the foreign donations of Tamiflu to Vietnam were confiscated by its army, which refused to share even with veterinarians working directly with infected flocks.[305]

But this appalling lack of vaccine and antivirals is not the only problem faced by the global "steerage class." The death tolls during the 1957 and 1968 pandemics were dramatically reduced by the widespread availability of new, effective antibiotics to treat secondary bacterial pneumonias—but the major bacterial pathogens, including the pneumococci and *H. influenzae,* have evolved resistance to penicillins erythromycin and other antibiotics usually employed in hospitals. Such a cycle of resistance is the inevitable result of natural selection, and the only solution is the constant development of new antimicrobial therapies, but the pharmaceutical industry has largely abandoned antibiotic research (although it sells huge quantities of antibiotics to the livestock industry and thus contributes to the accelerated obsolescence of the current generation of antibiotics). In the event of a pandemic, there is a great risk that mortality from bacterial pneumonia, especially in poor countries with limited supplies of older antibiotics, might return to pre–World War II levels. In July 2004 the Infectious Diseases Society of America issued a major white paper on the antibiotic crisis whose succinct punch line was "Bad bugs, no drugs."[306]

How would almost defenseless Third World cities respond

to a pandemic? The precedent that scares many public-health experts was the September 1994 outbreak of pneumonic plague in Surat, India's twelfth largest city. Laurie Garrett and, at greater length, Ghanshyam Shah have both discussed the Surat experience "as a warning of epidemics to come." A city of textile and diamond-cutting sweatshops and slums with one toilet for every 150 people, Surat epitomized the polarized condition of urban health care in most of the Third World: a small modern sector existed for the affluent, and a wretched mixture of inadequate public medicine and sheer quacksterism sufficed for the rest of the population.

Shah describes a "public health system [that] has not only gone downhill in its delivery system but also lost credibility. Even the poor do not trust it." Although Surat had no shortage of doctors, most of them were in private practice, "motivated by a quick profit. Ethical values among medical professionals are disappearing very fast."[307] As patients began to present plague symptoms, the doctors were the first to flee the plague. "They were totally unprepared for what followed. The private doctors panicked. Eighty percent of them fled the city, closing their clinics and hospitals and abandoning their patients. The fear in those physicians' eyes did not go unnoticed by the populace, and rumors of a great impending disaster spread swiftly among the largely illiterate masses. Surat's middle class discreetly packed their bags and slipped out of town."[308]

Within days, wild rumors had overrun India, antibiotic stocks had been depleted, and Delhi had been forced to send the elite Army Rapid Action Force to quarantine Surat's slum dwellers from fleeing in the footsteps of the middle classes.

The outside world, meanwhile, began to quarantine India, screening Indian jets or banning flights altogether; the Gulf states even stopped postal communications with the subcontinent. "WHO," Garrett writes, "did little to slow the [international] stampede toward hysteria or to stifle the opportunistic shouts of boycott." India appealed for international assistance, but few countries had inventories of plague vaccine, and new production would take six months.[309]

Fortunately the plague was contained in a week: "For many . . . a miracle," writes Shah. Experts debate whether the massive application of antibiotics (tetracycline and chloramphenicol) was decisive or whether the plague bacterium simply became less virulent through evolutionary modification. Nonetheless, the immediate explosion of panic, the desertion of private doctors, the hoarding of antibiotics, the absolute lack of confidence in government, the use of force to quarantine the poor, the silence of WHO Director-General Dr. Hiroshi Nakajima, and the hysterical stigmatization of India by its other countries—all confirmed experts' worse fears about the vicious circle of epidemic disease, slum poverty, and neoliberal politics.[310] An influenza pandemic would magnify the Surat experience perhaps a hundredfold.

The WHO is most worried about Africa. "Without a doubt, the virus will get there," Klaus Stohr told *Science* in October 2004. "The situation will be much, much worse than anywhere else. Access to vaccines will not be an option, let alone antivirals."[311] The 27 million or more Africans who are HIV positive, of course, would be the human bull's-eye of a H5N1 pandemic. "People with HIV/AIDS," says a CDC fact sheet, "are considered at increased risk from serious influenza-related complications. Studies have shown an increased risk for heart- and lung-related hospitalizations in people infected with HIV during influenza season . . . and a higher risk of influenza-related death."[312] AIDS, in other words, might become influenza's deadly dancing partner like malnutrition in India or malaria in Iran in 1918; as a result, the potential death toll could be a full order of magnitude higher than the estimated 2 million Africans killed by the 1918 pandemic. Yet, apart from some public notice taken in South Africa, the continent is wholly unprepared to address a pandemic; many countries do not even return influenza questionnaires to the WHO. (In many cases, public-health systems have simply collapsed under the relentless weight of AIDS and civil war.) World indifference towards the AIDS holocaust in Africa, moreover, provides a lamentable template for current global inaction in the face of the avian influenza threat.

13

Year of the Rooster

We're living on borrowed time.

Klaus Stohr (WHO)[313]

The Year of the Rooster, 2005, began with several more flu deaths in Vietnam. In two cases, the virus was contracted from eating raw duck blood pudding, a local delicacy savoured on ceremonial occasions. Tests showed that GenZ was now endemic amongst the hundreds of thousands of ducks and geese that roam Vietnamese farmyards that are in constant contact with chickens, pigs, and children. Because duck influenza is generally asymptomatic, there was no obvious way—apart from time-consuming and expensive blood testing—to distinguish infected from non-infected birds. Vietnam's desperate efforts at containment through the selective slaughter of poultry were undermined by the emergence of this "silent reservoir." Disoriented local authorities, as a result, grasped at questionable expedients. As the Vietnamese New Year approached, riot police set up checkpoints around Ho Chi Minh City to interdict the expected influx of infected poultry during Tet celebrations.[314] Municipal officials on 1 February also ordered the slaughter of all ducks in the city: a move that Dutch influenza expert Jan de Jong denounced as "really nonsense." He told an American reporter that the only way to stop the outbreak in Vietnam was "a near-total culling of the region's poultry and curtailment of poultry farming for several years."[315]

Hanoi retorted with justice that it needed more international aid to bolster its surveillance network and to compensate peasants whose flocks were being culled. The country was too poor to afford the destruction of a vital part of its subsistence economy without compensation from the richer nations for whom it was expected to provide an epidemic firewall. Foreign influenza experts working in Vietnam echoed Agriculture Minister Cao Duc Phat's appeal on 2 February for truly serious international assistance. Writing in the *New York Times*, Anton Rychener (the outspoken FAO representative in Vietnam), and Hans Troedsson (his WHO counterpart), pointed out that if the H5N1 outbreak had occurred in a poorer European country, there would have been a vast outpouring of money and medicine. "In the case of Asia, the international community has failed to come forward with enough money to finance desperately needed public health and veterinary measures and research on vaccines."[316] In an earlier interview with *Nature*, Dr. Jeremy Farar of Oxford University's clinical research unit in Ho Chi Minh City had lashed out at the dilettantish behavior of Western scientists: "When there's a problem, everyone flies in, creates a certain amount of havoc, flies out, and leaves nothing behind to change the situation." (He specifically exempted St. Jude's researchers and the crack Hong Kong team from his criticism.)[317] Incredibly, part of the shortfall of aid was most likely due to lobbying by Western poultry interests. With the Bush administration obviously in mind, *Nature* had editorialized in mid-January against the "mindset of protectionism" that obstructed veterinary aid to Vietnam. "Rich governments are disinclined to build up poor countries' ability to keep track of animal viruses, seeing this as economic assistance rather than humanitarian aid."[318]

Although the tsunami catastrophe in the Indian Ocean was the principal agenda item at the WHO executive board meeting on 25 January, the deteriorating flu situation in Vietnam was also on many minds. The Secretariat had circulated a briefing on pandemic preparedness that warned that the "present situation may resemble that leading to the 1918 pandemic." The report emphasized that "changes in the ecology of the disease and behavior of the virus have created multiple opportunities for a pandemic virus to emerge," and that gradual genetic drift, rather than reassortment, might be sufficient to unleash H5N1 on humanity. The Secretariat, underlining the "unprecedented opportunity to enhance preparedness," worried that vaccine development had not advanced "with a speed appropriate to the urgency of the situation."[319]

Some of the rich countries represented on the thirty-two-member executive board, however, were seemingly more concerned to protect pharmaceutical industry profits than to increase the availability of vaccines and antivirals. When Thai delegate Dr. Viroj Tangcharoensathien proposed (with the precedent of AIDS medications in mind) that the poor countries on the frontline of the avian flu battle be allowed to override drug patents in order to produce affordable quantities of Tamiflu, the American and French delegates vehemently objected and ultimately forced the meeting to adjourn without a vote. Dr. Anarfi Asamoa-Baah, the head of the WHO's communicable disease division, gloomily noted that "as a global community we are still ill prepared—and as long as one of us is not prepared, none of us is prepared."[320]

At a conference in Ho Chi Minh City a month later, this "alarming lack of commitment" from Japan, Europe, and the United States was again a top agenda item as Asian health officials responded to a warning by the WHO's Omi that the region was facing "the gravest possible danger of a flu pandemic." Shocked conferees heard one researcher after another outline fatal flaws in the underfunded avian flu surveillance system. The Japanese National Institute of Infectious Disease, which had retested blood samples from the Pasteur Institute in Ho Chi Minh City, reported that some of the negative results were in fact positive: suggesting that avian influenza, although perhaps not as lethal as suggested by confirmed cases, was actually more widespread and thus statistically closer to reassortment with human influenza. For its part, the Oxford University team in Ho Chi Minh City added fuel to the fire with a case-study of a four-year-old whose GenZ infection imitated acute encephalitis without respiratory symptoms. (Decades earlier, some scientists had associated a strange epidemic of sleeping sickness, *encephalitis lethargica*, with the 1918 H1N1 virus.) How many other similar cases had been misdiagnosed? Disturbingly, the child's stools were also full of H5N1—a warning that avian flu, like SARS two years before, might spread via poor sanitation. There was also nervous discussion of "insect vectors" after a startling announcement by Japanese researchers that they had found H5N1 in flies following the 2004 poultry outbreak.[321]

The gravest concern, however, was focused on the first flu deaths in Cambodia, a country with a corrupt government, primitive health services ($3 per capita annually), and no facility for the sophisticated serological analysis required to identify GenZ. Indeed, the outbreak only came to light when twenty-four-year-old Tit Sokan from Kampot province sought treatment in Vietnam.

Earlier, her fourteen-year-old brother had died after Cambodian doctors threw up their hands at his condition. "He had a fever and couldn't breathe normally so we took him to the hospital. The doctors gave him two bags of saline solution, then they told us to take him home. They said maybe we'd done something to offend our ancestors, and we should make an offering to them." Tit Sokan herself was too ill to be saved by antivirals, and after her death WHO investigators learned of border villages full of sick pigs and infected chickens. (In mid-April, another young woman from the same province died of suspected bird flu.)[322]

At the beginning of March, evidence was emerging of a second human-to-human transmission: this time in a Hanoi hospital where two nurses attended a critically ill avian flu patient, and both nurses developed the infection. Warning of the "perfect storm now gathering," *The Lancet* urged the European members of WHO to help Vietnam shut down small-scale free-range poultry production. "If the greatest pandemic in history is indeed on the horizon, that threat must be met by the most comprehensive public-health plan ever devised. That plan presently does not exist."[323] Meanwhile influenza authorities like Albert Osterhaus (University of Rotterdam) and Nancy Cox (CDC) were pleading in the pages of *Science* for the big Western labs to help Vietnam organize a broader, more accurate testing program in response to the troubling "information gap" about the evolution of GenZ.[324]

Researchers were appalled that the bird flu containment campaign in Vietnam was collapsing for lack of relatively trivial financial aid. Yet even on the U.S. home front, where "biosecurity" was supposedly a top priority, the CDC's budget for emergency public-health assistance was slashed by an eighth in fiscal

2005. Although plenty of money was found to increase funding for "abstinence education" (now $193 million per year), child immunization was reduced and preventive-health block grants to the states were eliminated. (A $20 million increase for pandemic vaccine hardly offset the loss of the block grants.) At a time of maximum menace, the CDC altogether lost $500 million in critical funding: a recession that only deepened gloom in an agency suffering, according to top official Robert Keegan, from a "crisis of confidence" that had led to the resignation of a score of top scientists and administrators. In an internal memo revealed by the *Washington Post* in March, Keegan spoke darkly of an "atmosphere of fear" and staff "cowed into silence" in the face of Director Julie Gerberding's autocratic style and her subservience to the administration's ideological agenda. Another CDC official described life in the agency as an "Alice in Wonderland environment where the CDC director is like the Queen of Hearts. You know, 'Off with their heads,'"[325] Meanwhile, an open revolt had broken out against the War on Terrorism's deleterious impact on university-based communicable disease research. Led by two Nobel prize-winners, 758 researchers signed a petition claiming that Washington's obsession with exotic but potentially weaponizable viruses and bacteria had resulted in a 27 percent decline in federal grants for research on tuberculosis and other major non-terror diseases.[326]

With this dissension in the background, Mike Leavitt, the new secretary of HHS, spoke to the National Academy of Sciences on 7 April about his department's strategy for dealing with H5N1. Following on the heels of an unexpected admission by Dr. Anthony Fauci, director of the National Institute of Allergy and Infectious Disease, that a flu pandemic was a greater immediate threat than a bioterrorist attack, Leavitt emphasized that avian influenza had the administration's full attention and that he was receiving daily briefings on the worrisome situation in Asia. He told his scientific audience that an H5N1 vaccine was in the human test stage, and that he had signed a $97 million contract with Sanofi Pasteur to develop new cell-based vaccine production lines.[327]

But the former governor of Utah did not address the problems inherent in vaccine production—the minuscule scale of the start-up, the long lead times, and the uncertainty whether current templates would match the evolved genome of a pandemic—that CDC Director Julie Gerberding had acknowledged in February at the annual meeting of the American Association for the Advancement of Science. Gerberding—according to a University of Minnesota news source—had warned that it was "nearly impossible to stop an outbreak by quarantining sick people" and "that flu vaccine production remains focused on ordinary seasonal flu, and it would be impossible to switch gears quickly to make a pandemic vaccine."[328] Leavitt also sidestepped widespread complaints about Washington's failure to stockpile Tamiflu in quantities comparable to recent purchases by Great Britain (14.6 million courses) and France (13 million).[329] Nor did he explain why the Bush administration was refusing to provide the aid that Vietnam so desperately needed to keep H5N1 in check.

Moreover, Leavitt's sunny assurances that Washington had public biosafety well in hand were immediately undercut by the startling revelation that a Cincinnati bioscience firm had sent out more than 5,000 samples of a deadly pandemic strain of influenza. H2N2, the "Asian flu" virus that killed 1 to 4 million people during the 1957 pandemic, had not circulated amongst humans since 1968 and was a grave threat to anyone born afterward. Influenza researchers, chastened by the escape of an earlier "lab fossil" (a strain of H1N1—the 1918 virus) in 1977, had long fretted about the security of H2N2 specimens in lab archives. They were incredulous that Meridian Bioscience—a contractor to the College of American Pathologists (CAP)—had knowingly included H2N2 in the viral test kits routinely used to assess quality control in laboratories across the world. CAP had not been informed of the strain's identity (which was, in any event, mislabeled on customs forms as "H3N2"), and most of the kits had been shipped through the U.S. mail. Although CDC experts had earlier urged the reclassification of H2N2 as a biosecurity level 3 agent, requiring the most stringent lab precautions, the recommendation was never implemented. As a result, "the CDC [did] not have regulatory authority over the distribution of the A (H2N2) influenza virus because it is not classified as a dangerous agent relevant to bioterrorism."[330]

Indeed, it was only thanks to Canadian vigilance that the pandemic threat was discovered at all. At the end of March, the National Microbiology Laboratory in Winnipeg identified H2N2—a strain the Canadians consider too dangerous to use in lab certification tests—in a patient sample sent from British Columbia. Although the Vancouver woman didn't actually have the flu, the contaminated sample was sufficient grounds for worldwide alarm. While Director Gerberding misleadingly reassured the public that "this strain of virus poses a very very low risk of transmission," the CDC mounted a frantic campaign to track down and destroy the thousands of samples.[331] A few missing test kits in Lebanon, near the epicenter of the Bush administration's fears about bioterrorism, caused considerable anxiety until they were finally accounted for by local labs. Like the Chiron scandal the year before, the H2N2 fiasco demonstrated the public peril of lax federal regulation of production protocols and biosafety standards. How could Washington pretend to defend the nation against the avian flu threat or bioterrorism, when it had allowed a private company to put a potential pandemic in the mail?

While the CDC was chasing the missing H2N2 samples, a joint summit in Paris of experts from the FAO and the OIE was reviewing the campaign against H5N1. Their sobering conclusion was that the virus had become too ecologically entrenched, particularly amongst asymptomatic ducks, to justify the continued economic and ethical costs of culling yet millions more domestic birds. Avian flu, in short, was endemic and inextinguishable. It was also utterly unpredictable: the discovery of a highly pathogenic H7 strain in North Korea in March raised fears of a doomsday recombination with "H5 lethality and H7 transmissibility." Meanwhile, the normally hermetic North Koreans clamored for international assistance to save their fledgling poultry export industry.[332]

As an alternative to the failed culls, the FAO and OIE proposed an ambitious poultry vaccination campaign in affected countries. The plan was a disappointment to experts who advocated the radical elimination of free-range poultry and wet markets. It also faced the formidable technical challenge of how to distinguish between vaccinated and infected birds, since their antibodies would otherwise be identical. More dauntingly, vaccination would require major financial aid to poor countries like Vietnam, Cambodia, and North Korea: "economic subsidies" likely to be opposed by corporate poultry producers and U.S.

conservatives. Not surprisingly only a few countries (Japan, Germany, and the Netherlands) were immediately prepared to support the Paris plan with modest contributions.[333]

By late spring 2005, therefore, every biological weathervane was pointing in the direction of an imminent pandemic. The basic WHO assessment of the threat—an inevitable outbreak that could kill millions, even tens of millions—had been accepted by all leading players, including the Bush administration. The rest of the print media had finally caught up with the *New York Times*, and avian influenza was almost daily in the news. Yet a certain quotient of disaster fatigue was also apparent: influenza experts, after all, had been warning of a viral apocalypse since the original Hong Kong outbreak in 1997. Almost nine years later, less than one hundred people had died and the pandemic was still just a prediction. In the meantime, tens of millions had died from AIDS, malaria, and diarrhoeal diseases. Is it possible that the WHO had exaggerated the threat of H5N1?

Indeed, a very vociferous camp of skeptics (few of them actually virologists) argue that avian flu is merely a "theoretical threat" and there may be some molecular inhibition that ensures that H5N1 will never acquire facile transmissibility amongst humans. Certainly there is much puzzlement that a pandemic hasn't yet emerged, but there is little evidence for the existence of a "factor X" preventing H5N1's mutation into a mass murderer. Quite the contrary: a breathtaking (and perhaps dangerous) scientific experiment in August confirmed frightening affinities between the current avian virus and the 1918 strain that killed more than 1 percent of humanity in the fall of 1918.

After a decade of painstaking lab work using lung tissue samples retrieved from the corpses of 1918 victims, the team headed by Jeffery Taubenberger at the Armed Forces Institute of Pathology outside of Washington, D.C., succeeded in deciphering H1N1—1918's complete genome. The major missing link had been the code for the polymerase complex of three proteins (PA, PB1, PB2) that are essential to the replication of the virus's genes inside the nucleus of the host cell. They found evidence of active evolution in one of these internal proteins, PB1, with strong indications that its mutations were a decisive factor, together with a unique HA (hemagglutinin), in generating the hyper-virulence of the 1918 virus. Even more stunningly, they discovered that all eight of its genes were purely avian. This confirmed that the great killer had acquired human transmissibility through a series of simple mutations in strategic proteins (HA, PB1, and perhaps NS) rather than through a reassortment of avian and human genes in co-infected pig or person as traditionally believed.[334] This clearly implies that H5N1 may not, after all, have to mix genes with a human virus: it may acquire pandemic velocity through its own incremental evolution. "If 1918 happened like this," Dr. Michael Osterholm fretted to the *Wall Street Journal*, "why couldn't or shouldn't 2005 happen like this? These viruses are kissing cousins."[335]

Indeed, it may be halfway there already. The Taubenberger group shared their research with another team led by Terrence Tumpey at the CDC in Atlanta that immediately employed the new genomic map to re-create the 1918 virus via plasmid-based reverse genetics. This alien resurrection horrified some scientists, like one "biosecurity expert" who warned *Nature*, "[T]he risk that the recreated strain might escape is so high, it is almost a certainty. And the publication of the full genome sequence gives any rogue nation or bioterrorist group all the information they need to make their own version of the virus."[336] Although many Americans have some immunity to H1N1 because of flu shots or (if they were born before 1957) exposure to descendant strains, an AWOL 1918 virus would pose a catastrophic public health threat to poor countries without annual vaccination programs or access to antivirals. Nonetheless, Tumpey's Frankenstein-like experiment was authorized by the CDC's Julie Gerberding on the grounds that any risk was outweighed by the urgency of learning more about the molecular dynamics of avian influenza. (After many protests, Gerberding did nix a crazy plan to send samples of the 1918 virus to other labs by U.S. mail or FedEx.)[337]

In any event, Tumpey's Atlanta team soon found themselves staring at Medusa's head. Compared with all other known human influenzas, its pathogenicity was simply off the scale. When mice, for instance, were infected with the 1918 virus, they eventually produced *39,000* times more viral particles than a contemporary H1N1 strain ("Texas 1991") that was used as a control. The mice with the control infection recovered, while the 1918 strain killed 100 percent of infected rodents. Tumpey and his colleagues quickly confirmed Taubenberger's hypothesis that this monstrous killing power derived from the collaboration of hemagluttinin and polymerase proteins (additional research would soon implicate the "non-structural" protein NS as well). The 1918 HA—unlike other human hemagluttinins—doesn't require the presence of a special enzyme (the protese trypsin) in host cells for successful infection and is able to reach deep into the respiratory system, achieving exceptionally high concentrations in lung cells. Meanwhile, only a dozen or so amino acid substitutions seem to differentiate 1918's PB1 polymerase from the "consensus" composition of ordinary, benign wild bird influenzas.[338]

H5N1 is already exceptionally lethal, but how close is it to acquiring the mutations needed for pandemic transmissibility between humans? According to Dr. Anthony Fauci, the director of the National Institute of Allergy and Infectious Diseases and the Bush administration's appointed spokesperson (along with Gerberding) on avian influenza, "[T]he H5N1 virus has accumulated five of the ten changes in the encoded polymerase protein sequences that were found in the 1918 virus and are commonly found in human influenza viruses. This suggests that the H5N1 virus may be accumulating changes associated with an increased likelihood of human-to-human transmission."[339] How long would such mutational "drift" take? Perhaps several decades. Taubenberger and his team found evidence that crucial 1918 polymerase mutations had been "circulating in human influenza viruses as early as 1900": implicit reproof to those who argue that if H5N1 had the capacity to become pandemic, it would have done so by now.[340]

Skeptics, however, continue to adduce new evidence that they believe undermines the case for an eventual H5N1 pandemic. Some argue that the death rate of H5N1 has been grossly overstated and that the virus may have been circulating for decades. Others point to recent research that shows the cells in the human upper respiratory tract (where infections are easily transmitted by coughing or sneezing) lack the appropriate receptors for avian flu. Unfortunately, neither line of argument actually contravenes the possibility that H5N1 will become pandemic. On one hand, a large-scale study of blood samples from southern China by veteran researchers at the University of Hong Kong found no evidence whatsoever of mild, undiagnosed H5 infections in the population.[341] On the other hand, the much-cited research by Yoshihiro

Kawaoka and his colleagues at the Universities of Wisconsin and Tokyo provides valuable insight into why human-to-human transmission of H5N1 is exceedingly difficult, but does not exclude the possibility that the virus will acquire the ability to infect the upper respiratory tract. Indeed, those with the patience to read scientific fine print will discover that Kawaoka et al. acknowledge that this has already occurred in the case of an ephemeral 2003 Hong Kong strain of H5N1.[342] There is no reason to believe that such a mutation won't repeat, and until more solid experimental evidence arises to support the cause of skepticism, the balance of scientific opinion remains on the side of veteran researchers like Robert Webster, J. Peiris, and Yi Guan, who in February 2006 reiterated that "the likelihood of an H5N1 influenza pandemic seems high, and the consequences could be catastrophic."[343]

A flu pandemic, alas, is not a fate we can avoid. To recapitulate an earlier argument: Third World urbanization and the Livestock Revolution have fundamentally transformed influenza ecology and accelerated the evolution of novel strains. Moreover there are multiple pathways to a new catastrophe on the scale of 1918. As we have seen, several subtypes of H7 and H9, in addition to H5N1, are also slouching toward Bethlehem with bright prospects of producing pandemic offspring. All the major candidates, in addition, appear to be increasing their evolutionary fitness to spread rapidly through avian and mammalian species. The fifteen HPAI outbreaks since 2000, for instance, have killed or led to the culling of ten times as many birds as all earlier known outbreaks combined. ("We've gone from a few snowflakes to an avalanche," an Italian researcher told *Science*.)[344] Even if humanity miraculously dodged H5N1, we would soon be under threat from other virulent avian subtypes.

Conclusion

*"Is it the birds?" asked Jill. "Have the birds done
it?"*[345]

Daphne du Maurier

Lake Qinghai (Lake Kokonor on older maps) is the Chinese
counterpart to Utah's Great Salt Lake. Until the 1970s it was also
nearly as large, but the waters of its tributary rivers and creeks
have been diverted to irrigate hayfields that support the burgeon-
ing local franchise of the livestock revolution. Although there
has been broad criticism of unsustainable water use and rampant
overgrazing in Qinghai Province, officials have done little to arrest the shrinkage of the lake, which seems inexorably headed
toward an Aral Sea–like extinction. Yet as its waters contract and
grow more saline, it remains a major stopover for tens of thousands of bar-headed geese, great cormorants, and other migratory
birds en route to far-flung wintering grounds in the Danube es-
tuary, Lake Victoria, the Ganges delta, and Queensland.

In spring 2005, as the first edition of this book was at the
printers, geese on Qinghai's celebrated Bird Island suddenly began to behave spasmodically, collapse, and quickly die. Local
wildlife authorities recognized this sinister death dance from
news accounts of avian flu outbreaks in Hong Kong and Vietnam, and viral samples from the dead geese were confirmed as
H5N1. The plague rapidly spread through the lake's entire avian

population, killing thousands of birds of diverse species. One ornithologist called it "the biggest and most extensively mortal avian influenza event ever seen in wild birds."[346] Indeed, no one had previously suspected that influenza of any subtype could become so lethal to its ancient hosts.

Once again H5N1 had taken an unexpected evolutionary turn, and Chinese virologists were shocked by the virulence of the new strain: when mice were infected with the Qinghai virus, they died even quicker than when injected with GenZ, the variant currently killing people in Vietnam and Indonesia. Yet the response of high-level Chinese authorities to the biological conflagration at Lake Qinghai struck both international and domestic experts as dangerously lackadaisical. Guan Yi—one of the celebrated Hong Kong team who have been tracking H5N1 since 1997—was publically critical of his country's officials. "They have taken almost no action to control this outbreak. They should have asked for international support. These birds will go to India and Bangladesh and then they will meet birds that come from Europe."[347]

In a paper published in *Nature*, Guan Yi and his colleagues revealed that the Qinghai strain was most likely derived from officially unacknowledged incidences of avian flu amongst poultry and wild birds in southern China.[348] This confirmed suspicions, already inflamed by Internet rumors of unreported human deaths, that Chinese authorities had reverted to the old pattern of concealing outbreaks from the rest of the world, as in 2003 when they had dissimulated the nature and extent of the SARS epidemic. And just as SARS whistle-blowers had been sanctioned, Beijing retaliated against Yi Guan for his scientific honesty, temporarily shutting down one of his laboratories at

Shantou University.[349] The conservative Agriculture Ministry was armed with new powers over basic research while its own laboratories refused to share Qinghai samples with overseas experts working for the WHO. In an unusual editorial, *Nature* was prompted to condemn the "mixture of secrecy and parsimony" that passed for avian flu strategy in China.[350]

In the meantime, China announced an extraordinary plan in fall 2005 to vaccinate some 5 billion domestic ducks and chickens. Animal vaccination on this scale had never been attempted or even contemplated before, and some experts expressed anxiety that poor compliance with biosafety protocols might actually spread the virus (via chicken manure on the boots of the vaccinators, for instance) or that flawed vaccines might produce populations of birds carrying the infection without displaying any sickness. Both fears seemed punctually realized in early 2006 as avian flu outbreaks erupted across China, and researchers discovered widespread evidence of asymptomatic infections. Monitoring the live poultry markets in southern China, the indefatigable Guan Yi and his team discovered that one out of every hundred "healthy" birds was, in fact, a dangerous carrier of H5N1. They also found little evidence that vaccination had succeeded in immunizing a majority of the poultry being put on sale in urban markets. Probably as a result of these stealth infections amongst birds, 16 human cases (11 fatal) had been acknowledged in China by the end of March 2006, with most of them occurring in areas like Shanghai, without officially reported poultry outbreaks.[351]

While this largely invisible viral explosion was taking place in China, a new human epicenter of H5N1 infection was emerging in Indonesia. In mid-July 2005, health officials confirmed that a father and his two young daughters had died of bird flu in a wealthy suburb of Jakarta. Disturbingly, the family had no known contract with poultry, and panic erupted amongst their neighbors as the local press speculated about possible human-to-human transmission. Six more human deaths together with poultry outbreaks in 23 provinces were reported through the autumn, forcing Indonesian officials to acknowledge that avian flu had become endemic in their country.

With an estimated 1.3 billion chickens in 30 million backyards, as well as a public-health system that has never recovered from the 1997 financial crisis, Indonesia quickly became the focus of much worry. Unlike Vietnam and Thailand, where both human and bird infections have been contained, at least temporarily, by aggressive government action, Indonesia has been very ineffective in combating an outbreak that has killed several dozen people as it spreads across the world's largest archipelago. As a leading Jakarta-based researcher told me in February 2006, "[T]his is the only avian influenza–affected country without a systematic control program. Action to contain the outbreak amongst ducks and chickens is haphazard and procrastination abounds. For the last six months Indonesia has been the hot spot of the world but it seems as if that hasn't really caused a change in policy."[352]

But the dangerous situations in China and Indonesia were eclipsed by international alarm over the sudden spread of H5N1 across Eurasia and into Africa. Just as Guan Yi and others had predicted, the flocks from Lake Qinghai began to take flight in midsummer, bringing avian flu to birds on the outskirts of Lhasa and then to the Siberian capital of Novosibirsk. By October, H5N1 had reached wild bird nesting grounds along the Black

Sea littoral, and cases were reported in the Crimea (Ukraine), Turkey, Bulgaria, and Romania, as well as from nearby Greece, Macedonia, and Croatia. The Turkish hotspot was quickly squelched, only to flare up again in December. When poultry started dropping dead in Agri province near the Iraqi border, residents immediately appealed for help but the government delayed several weeks before investigating. In the meantime, H5N1 vaulted across Anatolia from Van to Ankara, even to the outskirts of Istanbul. Three children in a single family became the first H5N1 victims outside of southeast Asia. Acutely aware that its future admission to the European Union might be prejudiced by a failed response to the avian flu crisis, the Turkish government redoubled efforts to track the outbreaks and cull infected flocks.

The success of this Turkish campaign, however, was promptly countered by new outbreaks and human fatalities in Iraq and Azerbaijan, followed by poultry cases in Kazakhstan, Georgia, Iran, Jordan, Gaza, and Israel. In February a new epidemic in southern Russia along the Caspian Sea and the lower Volga Valley killed one-half million birds. Crows and seagulls that fed on the carcasses soon spread the infection far afield. "Both the crows and gulls fly around," complained a local veterinary expert, "and in effect what we got was a rainfall of infected bird droppings."[353]

Then, while WHO and OIE attention was still focused on the Caspian and the Middle East, scores of swans started dying on Germany's Baltic island of Ruegen. Other dead birds turned up in Sicily, Austria, Sweden, Slovenia, and ultimately Scotland, while France's gourmet poultry belt was threatened by an outbreak amongst domestic turkeys. Europe went mildly berserk. Bavaria temporarily banned poultry sales, Poland outlawed pigeon races, tourists cancelled visits to Turkey, the Dutch and Germans brought their poultry indoors, the Scots proposed more bird hunting, the EU forbade the import of feathers from Siberia, and chicken *cordon bleu* disappeared from many bistro menus. Avian influenza was the undocumented immigrant from hell, mocking all of Europe's recent, frenzied efforts to seal itself off from the poor world on its eastern and southern doorsteps.

European health ministries, moreover, responded as if the EU didn't exist. The recently established European Center for Disease Prevention and Control is long overdue, but it lacks the authoritative clout and surveillance capability of its U.S. prototype. In the absence of a common strategy for combating H5N1, each government has made an independent assessment of the peril and has responded accordingly. Blair's "Fortress U.K.," for example, takes the specter of a flu apocalypse so seriously that it has stockpiled millions of courses of antivirals and prepared the nation to be governed from "Cobra," the Cabinet's secret war room in Whitehall. In contrast, Berlusconi has reacted so lethargically that Italy will be lucky to have enough body bags, much less Tamiflu, if the pandemic occurs in the near future. With most of the world's influenza vaccine production lines, as well as the only plant currently producing Tamiflu, Europe has literal life-and-death power over the estimated two or three billion people who would likely contract a pandemic influenza. Yet the European Parliament has to debate or acknowledge this special responsibility; and few governments, even of the nominal Left, are prepared to contest the hegemony of giant pharmaceutical corporations over world health.

Nor have the wealthy countries, despite recent promises to increase aid, yet transferred the minimal scientific resources required to keep H5N1 on the radar screen as it invades Africa and South Asia. The almost simultaneous arrival of avian flu in Nigeria, Egypt, India (where 50,000 birds died within a few days), and Pakistan in early 2006—along with the disclosure of 100 or more previously unreported outbreaks in Burma—dramatically raised the ante. In the Nigerian case, much valuable time was lost when dying poultry at commercial farms near Kano in January were misdiagnosed as suffering from Newcastle disease. Since then, the infection has spread to the Niger delta in the south of the country, as well as to several of Nigeria's impoverished Sahelian neighbors. It is also possible that local hotspots may exist in southern Sudan (the vast Sudd marshes) and the East African great lake region, but there is little or no local surveillance capacity, and poor farmers, as elsewhere, are reluctant to report dead birds and risk the culling of their flocks. The WHO, accordingly, is braced for the nightmare likelihood that human infections in sub-Saharan Africa will proliferate for weeks or even months before official detection.[354]

Between fall 2005 and spring 2006, avian influenza had spread at startling velocity to bird populations in at least 30 new countries, with a worrisome human epicenter in Egypt as well as several deadly clusters in the Middle East and a hotspot in northwestern India. Many observers were puzzled by avian influenza's seemingly capricious geography, but some epidemiologists were almost admiring. "H5N1 is a more sophisticated search engine than Google," I was told by Rob Wallace, a University of California scientist who is modeling the dynamics of a potential pandemic. He argues that bird flu on the wing is rapidly "expanding both the epidemiological and evolutionary space for the emergence of a pandemic strain." "The WHO's announced strategy of saturating an outbreak center—say a rural region of Vietnam or Thailand—with Tamiflu means nothing if H5N1 operates worldwide. By changing the spatial scale at which it operates, influenza changes the mix of interventions that will be necessary to stop it." (Indeed if recent cases in Turkey, Azerbaijan, Iraq, and Nigeria had involved a pandemic strain, the WHO would have lost the battle at the outset, since too much time elapsed between outbreak and the first official response.)

Wallace and some other researchers, moreover, see a consistent environmental logic in the emergence and spread of H5N1 that corresponds both to the livestock revolution with its "cities of birds," discussed earlier, and to the global degradation of wetlands. As water is dammed and diverted from wetlands, usually to support irrigated agriculture, migratory birds likewise tend to flock to irrigation canals and wet fields where free-range domestic poultry, especially ducks, are apt to have frequent contact with their excreted viruses. As Wallace puts it, "The displacement of wildfowl into the ecological space of free-ranging domestic birds creates a powerful interface for viral emergence. If the livestock revolution has ramped up flu virulence, wetland degradation leads to more combustible ecologies of wild and domestic waterfowl."[355]

Recent research has shown, for example, that the most important variable in explaining the location of avian flu outbreaks in Thailand is not the concentration of chickens but of outdoor domestic ducks. "Wetlands used for double-crop rice production," Marius Gilbert and his colleagues concluded, "where free-grazing duck feed year around in rice paddies, appear to be a critical factor in Highly Pathogenic Avian Infection [HPAI] persistence and spread."[356] Meanwhile, Guan Yi's team has discovered H5N1 infections amongst otherwise healthy wild ducks in China's Poyang Lake on the eve of their annual migration, a finding that resolves the paradox that "dead birds don't fly." Presumably, asymptomatic ducks and perhaps geese are the long-distance conveyors of avian flu, while the dead swans that have terrified western Europe are merely the victims and grim sentinels.[357] (The surprising genetic stability of the Lake Qinghai strain in the course of its Eurasian expansion has been interpreted by WHO researchers as evidence of H5N1's probably permanent adaptation to "at least some species of migratory waterfowl.")[358]

H5N1's recent travel itinerary offers circumstantial evidence of a two-way transmission belt linking wild birds, free-range domestic fowl, and industrial poultry. The original Nigerian outbreak, for example, occurred in commercial poultry farms in the region of the Kano River Irrigation Project, a huge network of dams and canals that divert water from Hadejia-Jama'are Basin and the seasonally inundated floodplains of the Hadejia-Nguru Wetlands. As the wetlands have been drained to accommodate the water hunger of Nigerian farmers who grow rice and maize, migratory birds—the Hadejia-Nguru is considered a "key site for Anatidae [swans, geese, and ducks]"—have begun to favor irrigated fields where they intermix in unprecedented ways with domestic birds.[359] Such diversions of wild birds from natural wetlands to rice paddies, irrigated fields, and farm ponds, of course, are nearly universal, and where they coincide with industrialized poultry production such conditions may constitute an optimal ecology for HPAI outbreaks.

At least this was the conclusion of the pathbreaking report

commissioned by the United Nations Environment Programme and presented to the Avian Influenza Scientific Seminar in Nairobi in April 2006. The report ("Avian Influenza and the Environment") found that "intensive poultry operations along migratory wild bird routes are incompatible with protecting the health of ecosystems that birds depend upon. They also increase the risks of transfer of pathogens between migrating birds and domestic fowl." The report concluded that current " 'heroic efforts' to contain avian influenza by killing wild birds or destroying their habitats were strictly 'counterproductive,' " and, instead, a worldwide campaign was needed to restore wetlands and reduce dangerous concentrations of mono-cultural poultry.[360] But nothing, unfortunately, is less likely than an immense effort to reconstruct agriculture upon sustainable ecological and epidemiological principles.

It is more likely that global ecological disorder will continue to express itself in bizarre and unexpected derangements of inter-species relationships. There is chilling evidence, for example, that H5N1 may be finding new pathways to humans through our pets. Many avian flu experts, including Andrew Jeremijenko at the U.S. Naval Medical Research Unit in Jakarta, are worried about enigmatic cases in Vietnam, China, and especially Indonesia, where human infections cluster in family groups without obvious histories of recent contact with infected poultry. In late January 2006 Jeremijenko was investigating human outbreaks in Indramayu on Java—"[W]ith all the free-grazing ducks and rice paddies I knew this area was going to be a problem"—and almost by whim decided to take a viral sample from a sick kitten he found. The little cat tested positive for H5N1; moreover, it was infected by a strain with distinctive amino-acid mutations previously identified in human cases but not in infected poultry, thus raising the disturbing possibility that some humans might be contracting avian flu from cats feeding on diseased birds.[361]

Cats have long concerned researchers. In late 2004, following the detection of avian flu in dead cats near Bangkok, the well-known team headed by Albert Osterhaus at Erasmus University in Rotterdam demonstrated that cats, shedding H5N1 in both their sputum and feces, could directly infect other cats. Thai researchers in 2005 were shocked to discover that 25 percent of dogs and 7 percent of cats sampled in a village in one of the chief poultry districts had antibodies to H5N1, evidence of past or current infection. More recently, "veterinarians in both Indonesia and Iraq have reported the high incidence of sudden death in cats during poultry outbreaks of avian flu." H5N1 infections amongst cats have also been confirmed in Germany and Austria, causing considerable dismay amongst cat lovers and pet owners in Europe.[362]

Researchers currently debate whether these cat infections are an ominous new threat to humans or a "viral dead end" posing little public health danger. Albert Osterhaus and his colleagues recently argued in *Nature* that "apart from the role that cats may play in H5N1 transmission to other species, they also may be involved in helping the virus to adapt to efficient human-to-human transmission." Osterhaus's team criticized the WHO for downplaying the possible role of cats and for failing to issue guidelines about the importance of keeping felines indoors in areas of current infection. But the problem is as much one of resources as of scientific consensus. Frustrated animal-health officials at the FAO complained to *Nature* that they were already overwhelmed with the Herculean task of monitoring poultry and lacked resources to surveil possible H5N1 outbreaks amongst tens of millions of dogs and cats.[363]

Americans, now officially warned by HHS Secretary Mike Leavitt that H5N1 is likely to arrive before the end of 2006, thus can only expect the unexpected.[364] As in Eurasia and Africa, the migration of avian flu to the United States will pit Rob Wallace's "viral search engine," with its demonic talent for finding novel niches and epidemiological weak points, against a still unprepared and ill-equipped public health system. Avian influenza, of course, remains an extremely rare disease of humans, and we must hope that it stays that way, since early clinical trials of the H5N1 vaccine that Sanofi Pasteur is developing for the federal government have yielded dismal results, with only 54 percent of volunteers mobilizing an immune response even at dosage levels twelve times higher than normal.[365] A recent poll of medical experts by Carnegie Mellon University "gave a median estimate of a less than 1 percent chance that the United States will have adequate stockpiles of vaccines or antiviral drugs to prevent a pandemic within the next three years."[366]

As we await the inevitable arrival of H5N1, casting nervous glances at the ducks in the pond or our neighbor's cat, it is worthwhile to reflect on the extraordinary causal chain that seems to link dying wetlands, factory chickens, and radical poverty to our deepest apprehensions about the safety of our own beloved. In her classic gothic short story "The Birds" (1952), Daphne du Maurier offered an avian apocalypse as an allegory for a world disordered by total war and the advent of atomic terror. What is H5N1 trying to tell us about the state of our earth?

Avian Influenza Timeline

1918		H1N1 pandemic kills 40–100 million people
1931		first influenza virus (swine H1N1) isolated
1933		human influenza isolated (H1N1)
1944		first flu vaccine
1957		H2N2 pandemic
1968		H3N2 pandemic
1976		swine flu debacle
1977		H1N1 reappears (lab escape?)

OUTBREAK

1996		H5N1 isolated from goose in Guangdong
1997		H5N1 outbreak in Hong Kong farms and poultry markets
		18 human cases (6 fatal)
2001		poultry outbreaks in Hong Kong
2003		SARS pandemic
	(Feb)	3 H5N1 cases (2 fatal) in Hong Kong (family returned from Fujian)
	(Mar)	H7N7 outbreak in Netherlands (dozens of human cases; 1 fatal)

FIRST WAVE

2003	(fall)	unreported outbreaks in Asia
	(Dec)	H5N1 confirmed amongst poultry in S. Korea
2004	(Jan)	poultry outbreaks reported in Japan, Laos, and Cambodia; human deaths in Vietnam and Thailand
	(Feb)	poultry outbreaks in Indonesia and China
		H7N3 outbreak in British Columbia (2 confirmed human cases)

Avian Influenza Timeline

SECOND WAVE

2004	(summer)	new poultry outbreaks in Vietnam, Thailand, China, and Indonesia
	(Aug)	new fatalities in Vietnam
	(Sep)	probable human-to-human transmission and death in Thailand
	(Nov)	second wave reported contained

THIRD WAVE

2005	(Jan)	human cases in Vietnam
	(Feb)	first human case and death in Cambodia
	(June)	China reports wild bird outbreak at Lake Qinghai
	(July)	new human epicenter in Indonesia
		poultry outbreaks in Siberia

MIGRATION ACROSS OLD WORLD

2005	(Aug)	outbreaks amongst poultry and/or wild birds in Kazakhstan, Tibet, and Mongolia
		complete mapping of 1918 genome; re-created in lab
	(Oct)	poultry cases in Turkey, Romania, Ukraine, and Croatia
		outbreaks spreading across China
		new human case in Thailand
2006	(Jan)	deaths in Turkey
	(Feb)	deaths in Iraq
	(Mar)	human cases in Azerbaijan
	(April)	deaths in Egypt

Since Feb. 2006 H5N1 was reported in more than 30 countries including Germany, Scotland, Sweden, France, Israel, Nigeria, India, Pakistan, and Burma.

Notes

1. Hao Juikratoke quoted in Bryan Walsh, "A Sickness Spreads," *Time* (Asia) (11 October 2004).

2. Albert Camus, *The Plague*, translated by Stuart Gilbert (New York: A. A. Knopf, 1948), p. 38.

3. My account is a composite of "Human Transmission Possible," and "Fear Grips Village in Kamphaeng Phet," *Nation* (Bangkok) (29 September 2004); ThailandChats.com, 3 October 2004; Noppawan Bunluesilp, "Fear Stalks Village of Thai Bird Flu Victim," *Reuters* (4 October 2004); Connie Levett, "Tens of Millions of Fowl Have Been Slaughtered in the Effort to Eradicate the Disease," *Age* (4 October 2004); Walsh, "Sickness Spreads" and Debora MacKenzie, "Bird Flu Transmitted Between Humans in Thailand," *New Scientist* (28 September 2004). In one account the village name is given as Ban Mu 19.

4. Kumnuan Ungchusak et al., "Probable Person-to-Person Transmission of Avian Influenza A (H5N1)," *New England Journal of Medicine* 352, no. 4 (27 January 2005): p. 336.

5. Ibid., pp. 339–40.

6. Pete Davies, *The Devil's Flu* (New York: Henry Holt, 2000), p. 75.

7. The pioneering article is R. Slemons et al., "Type A Influenza Viruses Isolated from Wild Free-Flying Ducks in California," *Avian Diseases* 18 (1974): pp. 119–24.

8. Cited in Edwin Kilbourne, *Influenza* (New York: Plenum Medical Book, 1987), p. 243.

9. Toshihiro Ito and Yoshihiro Kawaoka, "Avian Influenza," in *Textbook of Influenza*, edited by Karl Nicholson, Robert Webster, and Alan Hay (Oxford: Oxford Univ. Press, 1998), pp. 126 and 129.

Notes

10. Alan Hampson, "Influenza Virus Antigens and 'Antigenic Drift,' " in *Influenza*, edited by C. Potter (Amsterdam: Elsevier, 2003), p. 49.

11. J. Taubenberger and A. Reid, "Archaevirology: Characterization of the 1918 'Spanish' Influenza Pandemic Virus," in *Emerging Pathogens*, edited by Charles Greenblatt and Mark Spigelman (Oxford: Oxford Univ. Press, 2003), p. 189.

12. Steven Frank, *Immunology and Evolution of Infectious Disease* (Princeton: Princeton Univ. Press, 2002), p. 205.

13. John Holland, "Replication Error, Quasispecies Populations, and Extreme Evolution Rates of RNA Viruses," in *Emerging Viruses*, edited by Stephen Morse (New York: Oxford Univ. Press, 1993), p. 213.

14. Robert Webster and William Bean Jr., "Evolution and Ecology of Influenza Viruses: Interspecies Transmission," in Nicholson, Webster and Hay, *Textbook*, p. 117.

15. Holland, "Replication Error," pp. 207–9.

16. G. Air, A. Gibbs, W. Laver, and R. Webster, "Evolutionary Changes in Influenza B Are Not Primarily Governed by Antibody Selection," *Proc. Natl. Acad. Sci.* 87, no. 10 (1990): pp. 3884–88.

17. Dorothy Crawford, *The Invisible Enemy: A Natural History of Viruses* (Oxford: Oxford Univ. Press, 2000), p. 92.

18. Taubenberger and Reid, "Archaevirology," p. 196.

19. Christopher Scholtissek, Virginia Hinshaw, and Christopher Olsen, "Influenza in Pigs and Their Role as the Intermediate Host," in Nicholson, Webster, and Hay, *Textbook*, p. 143.

20. Brian Murphy, "Factors Restraining Emergence of New Influenza Viruses," in Morse, *Emerging Viruses*, p. 240.

21. Mark Gibbs, John Armstrong, and Adrian Gibbs, "Recombination in the Hemagglutinin Gene of the 1918 'Spanish Flu,' " *Science* 293 (7 September 2001): pp. 1842–45.

22. Ervin Fodor and George Brownlee, "Influenza Virus Replication," in Potter, *Influenza*, p. 18.

23. J. Oxford et al., "Antiviral Activity of Oseltamivir Carbosylate Against a Human Isolate of the Current H5N1 Chicken Strain," poster 3839, InterScience Conference on Antimicrobial Agents and Chemotherapy, Washington, DC, 31 August 2004.

24. Jocelyn Kaiser, "Facing Down Pandemic Flu, the World's Defenses Are Weak," *Science* 306 (15 October 2004): p. 394.

25. Richard Webby and Robert Webster, "Are We Ready for Pandemic Influenzas?" in *Learning from SARS: preparing for the next disease outbreak*, edited by Stacey Knobler et al. (Washington, DC: National Academies Press, 2004), p. 208.

26. Karl Nicholson, "Human Influenza," in Nicholson, Webster, and Hay, *Textbook*, p. 221.

27. See historical discussion in Jonathan Nguyen-Van-Tam, "Epidemiology of Influenza," in Nicholson, Webster, and Hay, *Textbook*, pp. 181–84.

28. T. Reichert et al., "Influenza and the Winter Increase in Mortality in the United States, 1959–1999," *American Journal of Epidemiology* 160, no. 5 (1 September 2004): pp. 492–502.

29. Lower figure from DHHS, *Draft Pandemic Influenza Preparedness and Response Plan,* August 2004, p. 3; and higher from James Stevens et al., "Structure of the Uncleaved Human H1 Hemagglutinin from the Extinct 1918 Influenza Virus," *Science* 303 (19 March 2004): p. 1866.

30. B. Schoub, J. McAnerney, and T. Besselaar, "Regional Perspectives on Influenza Surveillance in Africa," *Vaccine* 20, Suppl. 2 (15 May 2002): p. S46.

31. Alan Hampson, "Epidemiological Data on Influenza in Asian Countries," *Vaccine* 17, Suppl. 1 (30 July 1999): pp. S19–S23.

32. Schoub, McAnerney, and Besselaar, "Regional Perspectives," p. S46.

33. Leon Simonsen, "The Global Impact of Influenza on Morbidity and Mortality," *Vaccine,* 17, Suppl. 1 (30 July 1999): pp. S3–S10; F. Karaivanova, "Viral Respiratory Infections and Their Role as a Public Health Problem in Tropical Countries (Review)," *African Journal of Medicine and Medical Science* 24, no. 1 (1995): pp. 1–7; and C. Wong et al., "Influenza-Associated Mortality in Hong Kong," *Clinical Infectious Diseases* 39, no. 11 (1 December 2004): p. 1611.

34. Shoub, McAnerney, and Besselaar, "Regional Perspectives," S45–46; and "Influenza Outbreak in the District of Bosobolo, DRC, Nov.–Dec. 2002," *Weekly Epidemiological Record* 13 (28 March 2003): pp. 94–96.

35. WHO, *Avian Influenza and Human Health: Report by Secretariat,* Geneva (8 April 2004): p. 1.

36. For an overview of origin debate, see John Barry, "The Site of Origin

of the 1918 Influenza Pandemic and its Public Health Implications," *Journal of Translational Medicine* 2, no. 3 (20 January 2004): pp. 1–4.

37. Niall Johnson and Juergen Mueller, "Updating the Accounts: Global Mortality of the 1918–1920 'Spanish' Influenza Pandemic," *Bulletin of the History of Medicine* 76 (2002): tables 1–5; and Edwin Oakes Jordan, *Epidemic Influenza* (Chicago: American Medical Association, 1927).

38. Ibid. pp. 108 and 115; and K. Davis, *The Population of India and Pakistan* (Princeton, NJ: Princeton Univ. Press, 1951), p. 37 (estimate of 20 million dead).

39. I. Mills, "The 1918–19 Influenza Pandemic—The Indian Experience," *Indian Economic and Social History Review* 23, no. 1 (1986): pp. 1–40.

40. Ibid., p. 35.

41. Mridula Ramanna, "Coping with the Influenza Pandemic: The Bombay Experience," in *The Spanish Influenza Pandemic of 1918–19: New Perspectives*, edited by Howard Phillips and David Killingray (London: Routledge, 2003), p. 95.

42. Quoted in Peter Harnetty, "The Famine That Never Was: Christian Missionaries in India, 1918–1919," *Historian* (Spring 2001): p. 2.

43. Ramanna, "Bombay Experience," p. 97.

44. Mills, "Indian Experience," pp. 34–35.

45. Johnson and Mueller, "Updating the Accounts," p. 106 (research of Svenn-Erik Mamelund).

46. Amir Afkhami, "Compromised Constitutions: The Iranian Experience with the 1918 Influenza Pandemic," *Bulletin of the History of Medicine* 77 (2003): pp. 371–72.

47. Ibid., pp. 386–91.

48. Kevin McCracken and Peter Curson, "Flu Downunder," in Phillips and Killingray, *Spanish Influenza*, pp. 130–31.

49. Memo, 15 March 1976, quoted in Richard Neustadt and Harvey Fineberg, *The Epidemic That Never Was* (New York: Vintage Books, 1982), p. 207.

50. John Barry, *The Great Influenza* (New York: Viking, 2004), p. 5.

51. J. Oxford et al., "World War I May Have Allowed the Emergence of 'Spanish' Influenza," *Lancet Infectious Diseases* 2, no. 2 (February 2002): pp. 11–14.

52. William Henry Welch, quoted in Alfred Crosby, *America's Forgotten*

Pandemic: The Influenza of 1918, new ed. (Cambridge: Cambridge Univ. Press, 2003), p. 11.

53. Jeffrey Taubenberger et al., "Integrating Historical, Clinical and Molecular Genetic Data in Order to Explain the Origin and Virulence of the 1918 Spanish Influenza Virus," *Phil. Trans. R. Soc. London* B 356 (2001): p. 1831.

54. National Academy of Sciences, "Thomas Francis Jr.," *Biographical Memoirs* 44 (Washington, DC: 1974), pp. 71–73.

55. Edwin Kilbourne et al., "The Total Influenza Vaccine Failure of 1947 Revisited," *PNAS* 99, no. 16 (6 August 2002): pp. 10748–52.

56. Gerald Pyle, *The Diffusion of Influenza: Patterns and Paradigms* (Totowa, NJ: Rowman & Littlefield, 1986), p. 141.

57. J. Donald Millar and June Osborne, "Precursors of the Scientific Decision-Making Process Leading to the 1976 National Immunization Campaign," in *Influenza in America, 1918–1976*, edited by Osborne (New York: Prodist, 1977), pp. 22–23.

58. Global mortality for 1957 pandemic from testimony of Anthony Fauci, Director of the National Institute of Allergy and Infectious Diseases, to the House Committee on Government Reform, 12 February 2004.

59. Miller and Osborne, "Precursors," pp. 21–23.

60. Ibid.; and 1968 global estimate from Fauci testimony.

61. Pyle, *Diffusion*, p. 141.

62. M. Kitler, P. Gavinio, and D. Lavanchy, "Influenza and the Work of the World Health Organization," *Vaccine* 20, Suppl. 2 (15 May 2002): p. 9, www.sciencedirect.com.

63. Miller and Osborne, "Precursors," pp. 19–22.

64. See the recollections by famed Australian influenza researcher Graeme Laver, "Influenza Virus Surface Glycoproteins, Haemagglutinin and Neuraminidase: A Personal Account," in Potter, *Influenza*, pp. 31–47.

65. Neustadt and Fineberg, *Never Was*, pp. 17–22.

66. Ibid., p. 35.

67. Ibid., pp. 64 and 81.

68. Ibid., pp. 67 and 95.

69. Kilbourne, *Influenza*, p. 331.

70. Ibid., p. xx.

71. Ibid., pp. 225–26.

Notes

72. Jaap Goudsmit, *Viral Fitness: The Next SARS and West Nile in the Making* (Oxford: Oxford Univ. Press), p. 23.

73. Edward Stokes, *Hong Kong's Wild Places* (Hong Kong: Oxford Univ. Press, 1995), pp. 175–76.

74. Davies, *Devil's Flu*, p. 2.

75. D. Alexander, "A Review of Avian Influenza in Different Bird Species," *Veterinary Microbiology* 74 (2000): pp. 3–13.

76. K. Shortridge, J. Peiris, and Y. Guan, "The Next Influenza Pandemic: Lessons from Hong Kong," *Journal of Applied Microbiology* 94, Symposium Supplement (2003): p. 71S.

77. Rene Sancken et al., "The Next Influenza Pandemic: Lessons from Hong Kong, 1997," *Emerging Infectious Diseases* 5, no. 2 (March–April 1999): p. 198.

78. Davies, *Devil's Flu*, pp. 8–12. Davies's vivid account, based on wide-ranging interviews and travel to Hong Kong, is preferred to Gina Kolata's error-ridden narrative, *Flu* (New York: Farrar, Straus, Ginoax 1999). Kolata, a *New York Times* science reporter who relies unduly on the CDC version of events, gets the date of the little boy's death wrong and, more significantly, fails to acknowledge that the Dutch were first to make the type identification.

79. Robert Webster and Alan Hay, "The H5N1 Influenza Outbreak in Hong Kong: A Test of Pandemic Preparedness," in Nicholson, Webster, and Hay, *Textbook*, p. 561.

80. Davies, *Devil's Flu*, p. 19; Jocelyn Kaiser, "1918 Flu Experiments Spark Concerns About Biosafety," *Science* 306 (22 October 2004): p. 591; and Agriculture Research Service, USDA, "Containing the Hong Kong Poultry Flu Outbreak," (December 1998), see www.ars.usda.gov.

81. Robin Ajello and Catherine Shepherd, "The Flu Fighters" (1998), Asiaweek.com.

82. Gretchen Reynolds, "The Flu Hunters," *New York Times Magazine*, 7 November 2004.

83. It is important to note, however, that researchers never found any direct evidence of the route of transmission: whether by contact with bird feces or direct inhalation of aerosolized virus. See Anthony Mounts et al., "Case-Control Study of Risk Factors of Avian Influenza A (H5N1) Disease, Hong Kong, 1997," *Journal of Infectious Diseases* 180 (1999): pp. 507–8.

Notes

84. Ajello and Shepherd, "Flu Fighters," p. 2.

85. Shortridge, Peiris, and Guan, "Next Influenza Pandemic," p. 72S.

86. Quoted in Goudsmit, *Viral Fitness*, p. 148.

87. Richard Krause, "Foreword," in Morse, *Emerging Viruses*, p. vii.

88. William McNeill, "Control and Catastrophe in Human Affairs," *Daedalus* 118, no. 1 (1989): pp. 1–12.

89. Ibid.

90. William McNeill, "Patterns of Disease Emergence in History," in Morse, *Emerging Viruses*, p. 33.

91. Justin Brashares et al. "Bushmeat Hunting, Wildlife Declines, and Fish Supply in West Africa," *Science* 306 (12 November 2004): pp. 1180–82.

92. "Bushmeat and the Origin of HIV/AIDS," conference abstract, Environmental and Energy Study Institute, Washington, DC, February 2002; and BBC news file, "AIDS Warning over Bushmeat Trade," 26 October 2004.

93. Yanzhong Huang, "The SARS Epidemic and its Aftermath in China: A Political Perspective," in Stacey Knobler, *Learning from SARS,* p. 127.

94. *Sidney Morning Herald*, 9 April 2003.

95. National Academy of Sciences, *Growing Populations, Changing Landscapes: Studies from India, China, and the United States* (Washington, DC: National Academy Press, 2001), pp. 211, 212, 214, and 220.

96. Ibid.

97. WHO press release, "Increased Surveillance for Influenza Should Be Continued," 28 January 1998.

98. Guo Yuanji, "Influenza Activity in China: 1998–1999," *Vaccine* 20, Suppl. 2 (15 May 2002): pp. 28–35.

99. K. Li et al., "Characterization of H9 Subtype Influenza Viruses from the Ducks of Southern China: a Candidate for the Next Influenza Pandemic in Humans?" *Journal of Virology* 77, no. 12 (June 2003): pp. 6988–89.

100. Simon Levin, "Population Biology and the Evolution of Influenza A," (working paper, n.d.), p. 23.

101. Li, "H9 Subtypes," pp. 6989 and 6992–93.

102. *New Scientist* interview quoted on eces.org/articles/00760.php.

103. K. Shortridge, "Next Influenza Pandemic," pp. 73–74.

104. Li, "H9 Subtypes," p. 6993.

105. K. Choi et al., "Continuing Evolution of H9N2 Influenza Viruses

in Southeastern China," *Journal of Virology* 78, no. 16 (August 2004): pp. 8609–14.

106. Yi Guan et al., "Emergence of Multiple Genotypes of H5N1 Avian Influenza Viruses in Hong Kong Special Administrative Region," *PNAS* 99, no. 13 (25 June 2002): p. 8950–54.

107. Emma Young, "Hong Kong Chicken Flu Slaughter 'Failed,'" *New Scientist*, 19 April 2002.

108. Katharine Sturm-Ramirez et al., "Reemerging H5N1 Influenza Viruses in Hong Kong in 2002 Are Highly Pathogenic to Ducks," *Journal of Virology* 78, no. 9 (May 2004): p. 4899.

109. Ibid., pp. 4892–4900.

110. "Update on the Avian Influenza Situation #26," *FAOAIDE News* (20 December 2004): p. 2.

111. Shortridge, Peiris, and Guan, "Next Influenza Pandemic," p. 77S.

112. J. Peiris et al., "Re-emergence of Fatal Human Influenza A Subtype H5N1 Diseases," *Lancet* 363 (21 February 2004): pp. 617–19.

113. "An Avian Flu Jumps to People," *Science* 299 (7 March 2003): p. 1504.

114. Robin Weiss and Angela McLean, "What Have We Learnt from SARS?" *Phil. Trans. R. Soc. Lond.* 359 B (2004): p. 1139.

115. WHO, "SARS: Chronology of a Serial Killer," Update 95; and Tabitha Powledge, "Genetic Analysis of Bird Flu," *Scientist*, 27 February 2003.

116. Huang in Knobler, *Learning from SARS*, p. 118.

117. J. Mackenzie et al., "The WHO Response to SARS and Preparations for the Future," in Knobler, *Learning from SARS*, p. 43; and Karen Monaghan, "SARS: Down But Still a Threat," in Knobler, *Learning from SARS*, p. 249 (CDC chart).

118. I. Yu and J. Sung, "The Epidemiology of the Outbreak of SARS in Hong Kong—What We Do Know and What We Don't," *Epidemiol. Infect.* 132 (2004): pp. 784: Hong Kong Department of Health, "Outbreak of SARS at Amoy Gardens, Kowloon Bay, Hong Kong: Main Findings of the Investigation," 17 April 2003.

119. "Summary and Assessment," in Knobler, *Learning from SARS*, p. 4.

120. Huang in Knobler, *Learning from SARS*, pp. 123–25.

121. Ibid.; also Monaghan in Knobler, *Learning from SARS*, p. 255.

122. Y. Guan et al., "Isolation and Characterization of Viruses Related to

Notes

the SARS Coronavirus from Animals in Southern China," in Knobler, *Learning from SARS*, pp. 157–65.

123. Diana Bell, Scott Roberton, and Paul Hunter, "Animal Origins of SARS Coronavirus: Possible Links with the International Trade in Small Carnivores," *Phil. Trans. R. Soc. Lond.* 359 B (2004): pp. 1107 and 1112.

124. Goudsmit, *Viral Fitness*, p. 142.

125. C. Naylor, Cyril Chantler, and Sian Griffiths, "Learning from SARS in Hong Kong and Toronto," *JAMA* 291, no. 20 (26 May 2004): pp. 2483–84. Also Abu Abdullah et al., "Lessons from the Severe Acute Respiratory Syndrome Outbreak in Hong Kong," *Emerging Infectious Diseases* 9, no. 9 (September 2003): p. 2 (on Chinese health workers).

126. Robert Webster, "Wet Markets—A Continuing Source of Severe Acute Respiratory Syndrome and Influenza?" *Lancet* 363 (17 January 2004): p. 236.

127. Roy Anderson et al., "Epidemiology, Transmission Dynamics and Control of SARS: The 2002–2003 Epidemic," *Phil. Trans. R. Soc. Lond*, 359 B (2004): p. 1104.

128. Goudsmit, *Viral Fitness*, p. 148.

129. J. Peiris and Y. Guan, "Confronting SARS: A View from Hong Kong," *Phil. Trans. R. Soc. Lond*, 359 B (2004): p. 1077.

130. Anderson, "Transmission Dynamics," p. 1096.

131. Weiss and McLean, "What Have We Learnt?" p. 1139.

132. Quoted in Bernice Wuethrich, "Chasing the Fickle Swine Flu," *Science* 299 (7 March 2003): p. 1502.

133. For the evidence that implicates Kansas, see Barry, "The Site of Origin."

134. Christopher Delgado, Mark Rosegrant, and Nikolas Wada, "Meating and Milking Global Demand: Stakes for Small-Scale Farmers in Developing Countries," in *The Livestock Revolution: A Pathway from Poverty?* edited by A. Brown (Canberra ATSE Crawford Fund, 2003), p. 17, tables 4–5; and FAO Statistics Database.

135. Ibid., p. 14.

136. UNEP/GEF, "Protecting the Environment from the Impact of the Growing Industrialization of Livestock Production in East Asia," working paper, Phuket (Thailand) 2003, p. 1.

201

Notes

137. Donald Stull and Michael Broadway, *Slaughterhouse Blues: The Meat and Poultry Industry in North America* (Belmont, CA: Thompson/Wadsworth, 2004), p. 41.

138. James Rhodes, "The Industrialization of Hog Production," *Review of Agricultural Economics* 17 (1995): pp. 107–18.

139. William Boyd and Michael Watts, "Agro-industrial Just-in-Time: The Chicken Industry and Postwar American Capitalism," in *Globalising Food: Agrarian Questions and Global Restructuring*, edited by Michael Goodman and Michael Watts (London: Routledge, 1997), p. 209.

140. J. van Middelkoop, "High Density Broiler Production—The European Way," Government of Alberta Poultry Website, www.agric.gov.ab.ca./livestock/poultry.

141. Ron Fouchier et al., "Avian Influenza A Virus (H7N7) Associated with Human Conjunctivitis and a Fatal Case of Acute Respiratory Distress Syndrome," *PNAS* 101, no. 5 (3 February 2004): p. 1360.

142. Marion Koopmans et al., "Transmission of H7N7 Avian Influenza A Virus to Human Beings during a Large Outbreak in Commercial Poultry Farms in the Netherlands," *Lancet* 363 (21 February 2004): p. 587.

143. Ibid., pp. 587–88.

144. Ibid., pp. 588–90; Adam Meijer et al., "Highly Pathogenic Avian Influenza Virus A (H7N7) Infection of Humans and Human-to-Human Transmission during Avian Influenza Outbreak in the Netherlands," in *Options for the Control of Influenza V*, edited by Y. Kawaoka (Amsterdam, Elsevier, 2004), pp. 65–68; Martin Enserink, "Bird Flu Infected 1000," *Science* 306 (22 October 2004): p. 590; and Fox News, "Dutch Investigation Shows Bird Flu Outbreak Worsens in the Netherlands," 18 January 2005 (2000 figure).

145. Enserink, "Bird Flu," p. 590.

146. Fouchier, "Avian Influenza A," p. 1360.

147. Koopmans, "Transmission of H7N7," p. 593.

148. Wuethrich, "Fickle Swine Flu," pp. 1502–5; and Christopher Olsen, Gabriele Landolt, and Alexander Karasin, "The Emergence of Novel Influenza Viruses among Pigs in North America due to Interspecies Transmission and Reassortment," in Kawaoka, "Options," pp. 196–98.

149. Rodger Ott quoted in Wuethrich, "Fickle Swine Flu," p. 1503.

150. Wuethrich, "Fickle Swine Flu," p. 1503.

151. P. Woolcock, D. Suarez, and D. Kuney, "Low-Pathogenicity Avian Influenza Virus (H6N2) in Chickens in California, 2000–02," *Avian Diseases* 47, Suppl. 3 (2003): pp. 872–81.

152. "Summary and Assessment," in *The Threat of Pandemic Influenza: Are We Ready?*, edited by Knobler et al. (Washington D.C.: Institute of Medicine 2005), pp. 21–23.

153. Ibid.

154. Carol Cardona, "Low Pathogenicity Avian Influenza Outbreaks in Commercial Poultry in California," in Knobler, *Threat*, p. 195.

155. For a review of the debate, see D. Alexander, "Should We Change the Definition of Avian Influenza for Eradication Purposes?" *Avian Diseases* 47, Suppl. 3 (2003): pp. 976–81.

156. Jim Monke, "Avian Influenza: Multiple Strains Cause Different Effects Worldwide," Congressional Research Service, Report for Congress (14 May 2004), pp. 3–5, and USDA, see www.aphis.usda.gov.

157. Canadian Broadcasting Corporation, 8 November 2004.

158. Martin Hirst et al., "Novel Avian Influenza H7N3 Strain Outbreak, British Columbia," *Emerging Infectious Diseases* 10, no. 12 (December 2004).

159. S. Tweed et al., "Human Illness from Avian Influenza H7N3, British Columbia," *Emerging Infectious Diseases* 10, no. 12 (December 2004): pp. 1–2 (CDC Website edition).

160. Ibid., p. 4.

161. CBC News, "Federal Agency Accused of Mishandling Avian Flu in B.C.," 19 January 2005.

162. Wuethrich, "Fickle Swine Flu," p. 1505.

163. Jasper Becker, "Bird Flu Hits China," *Independent* (London), 30 January 2004.

164. A. Fumihito et al., "One Subspecies of the Red Junglefowl (Gallus gallus gallus) Suffices as the Matriarchic Ancestor of all Domestic Breeds," *PNAS* 91 (20 December 1994): pp. 12505–9.

165. Christopher Delgado, Clare Narrod, and Marites Tiongco, "Policy, Technical, and Environmental Determinants and Implications of the Scaling-Up of Livestock Production in Four Fast-Growing Developing Countries: A Synthesis," (IFFPRI/FAO working paper, 2003), section 2.2, "Growth and Concentration in Thailand."

Notes

166. See www.cpthailand.com.

167. Isabelle Delforge, "The Flu That Made Agribusiness Stronger," originally published in *Bangkok Post*, posted at www.focusweb.org.

168. Felicity Lawrence, "Fowl Play," *Guardian*, 8 July 2002.

169. William Roenick, "World Poultry Consumption," *Poultry Science* 78 (1999): pp. 722–28.

170. Erick Stowers, "Chinagate Scandal," *Pressing Times*, Spring 2002.

171. Dan Moldea and David Corn, "Influence Peddling, Bush Style," *Nation* (New York), 23 October 2000.

172. Pasuk Phongpaichit, *Corruption, Governance, and Globalisation: Lessons from the New Thailand*, Corner House Briefing #29 (London 2003), p. 18.

173. Bruce Einhorn, "China: New Plague, Same Coverup?" *BusinessWeek Online* (10 February 2004)

174. "Bird Flu Found in Smuggled Duck," *Taipei Times*, 1 January 2004.

175. Debora MacKenzie, "Bird Flu Outbreak Started a Year Ago," *New Scientist*, 28 January 2004.

176. Robin McKie et al., 'Warning as Bird Flu Crossover Danger Escalates," *Observer*, 12 December 2004.

177. Senator Nirun Phitakwatchara, quoted in "Thailand and Cambodia Admit Bird Flu," *New Scientist*, 23 January 2004.

178. *Bangkok Post* (30 January, 5–6 February, and 25 March), quoted in Isabelle Delforge, "Thailand: The World's Kitchen," *Le Monde diplomatique* (English edition), July 2004.

179. Anton Rychener, the FAO representative in Hanoi, told the press in February 2004 that Vietnamese poultry had been testing positive for avian flu "for months." See Keith Bradsher, "Bird Flu Is Back," *New York Times*, 30 August 2004.

180. Justin McCurry, "Bird Flu Suicides in Japan," *Guardian*, 9 March 2004.

181. Quoted in *Bangkok Post*, 7 February 2004.

182. David Cyranoski, "Vaccine Sought as Bird Flu Infects Humans," *Nature* 422 (6 March 2003).

183. Richard Ehrlich, "Thailand Denies Bird Flu Cover-Up" (26 January 2004), www.scoop.co.nz.

184. "Cover-up Began Last Year," *Nation* (Bangkok), 23 January 2004; and *Manager* (2 February 2004), cited in Chanida Chanyapate and Isabelle

204

Delforge, "The Politics of Bird Flu in Thailand" (19 April 2004), www.focusweb.org.

185. "Thai PM Admits Mistakes Over Bird Flu," *Guardian Unlimited*, 28 January 2004.

186. Sirima Manapornsamrat, quoted in "Thailand's Poultry Industry Facing Huge Losses from Bird Flu Crisis" (25 January 2004), www.eubusiness.com.

187. "Sukhothai Death: Victims of the Information Gap," *Nation* (Bangkok), 2 February 2004.

188. Interviewed by Delforge, "Thailand: The World's Kitchen."

189. Ibid.

190. "Chicken Exports: Watana Threatens Retaliation," *Nation* (Bangkok), 4 February 2004.

191. Chanyapate and Delforge, "Politics,"

192. FAO press release, Bangkok, 28 January 2004.

193. Slingenbergh et al., "Ecological Sources of Zoonotic Diseases," *Rev. Sci. Tech. Off. Epiz.* 23, no. 2 (2004): p. 476.

194. Delforge, "The Flu," and "Hay Tay Wages Grueling War on Avian Flu," *Vietnam News*, 4 February 2004.

195. John Aglionby, "The Politics of Poultry," *Guardian*, 29 January 2004.

196. Leu Siew Ting, "China: Criticism Grows Over Media Coverage," *South China Morning Post*, 11 February 2004.

197. Chanyapate and Delforge, "Politics," "Focus on Foreign Wildfowl," *Nation* (Bangkok), 26 January 2004; and "Pigeons to Be Slaughtered," *Nation* (Bangkok), 30 January 2004.

198. Secretariat, WHO, "Avian Influenza and Human Health," Geneva (8 April 2004); and Keith Bradsher and Lawrence Altman, "A War and a Mystery: Confronting Avian Flu," *New York Times*, 12 October 2004.

199. Associated Press, 1 February 2004.

200. "China: Towards 'Xiaokang,' but Still Living Dangerously," *Lancet* 363 (7 February 2004): p. 409.

201. Webster, "Wet Markets," pp. 234–36.

202. Y. Guan et al., "H5N1 influenza: A Protean Pandemic Threat," *PNAS* 101, no. 20 (25 May 2004): pp. 8156–57.

203. Ibid.

204. Alison Abbott and Helen Pearson, "Fear of Human Pandemic Grows as Bird Flu Sweeps through Asia," *Nature* 427 (5 February 2004): pp. 472–73.

205. Joint statement by FAO and OIE, 23 March 2004.

206. Quoted in Keith Bradsher and Lawrence Altman, "UN Health Official Foresees Tens of Millions Dying in a Global Flu," *New York Times*, 29 November 2004.

207. Reuters, "US Chicken Exports Rise," 28 January 2004; notes at www.thaistocks.com; "Bird-flu Outbreaks Elsewhere Present Opportunities to Taiwan Exporters," 23 February 2004, www.taiwanheadlines.gov.tw; and Delforge, "The World's Kitchen."

208. K. Li et al., "Genesis of a Highly Pathogenic and Potentially Pandemic H5N1 Influenza Virus in Eastern Asia," *Nature* 430 (8 July 2004): pp. 209–12.

209. Who, "Laboratory Study of H5N1 in Domestic Ducks," WHO press release, October 2004; and H. Chen et al., "The Evolution of H5N1 Influenza Viruses in Ducks in Southern China," *PNAS* 101, no. 28 (13 July 2004): p. 10452.

210. Li, "Genesis," pp. 209–12.

211. Jeffery Taubenberger, Ann Reid, and Thomas Fanning, "Capturing a Killer Flu Virus," *Scientific American* (January 2005): p. 70.

212. Reynolds, "Flu Hunter."

213. Report by the Secretariat, WHO, *Avian Influenza and Human Health*, Geneva (8 April 2004), p. 3.

214. David Cyranoski, "Bird Flu Data Languish in Chinese Journals," *Nature* 430 (26 August 2004): p. 955.

215. Donald McNeil, "Experts Call Wild Birds Victims, not Vectors," *New York Times*, 12 October 2004.

216. Shaoni Bhattacharya, "Three People Killed by Bird Flu in Vietnam," *New Scientist*, 12 August 2004.

217. WHO release, 12 September 2004, www.smh.com.au.

218. "Concern over Bird, Humanflu Outbreaks," *Nation* (Bangkok), 15 September, and "Bird Flu Suspected in Child Deaths," *Nation* (Bangkok), 24 September 2004.

219. "Cambodia: Outbreak of Bird Flu," *Nation* (Bangkok), 22 September 2004.

220. "Thailand Offers Chicken for Russian Arms," *Moscow News*, 1 September 2004.

221. Bryan Walsh, "Sickness Spreads," and Debora MacKenzie, "Bird Flu Transmitted between Humans in Thailand," *New Scientist*.

222. "Cabinet Given Bird-Flu Deadline," *Nation* (Bangkok), 30 September 2004.

223. "Young Girl becomes Third Bird Flu Fatality," *Nation* (Bangkok), 5 October 2004.

224. Thijs Kuiken et al., "Avian H5N1 Influenza in Cats," *Science* 306 (8 October 2004): p. 241.

225. Deborah MacKenzie, "Europe Has Close Call with Deadly Bird Flu," *New Scientist*, November 2004.

226. "Flu Pandemic 'Could Wreck Ecosystem,'" *Seven News* (Australia), 11 December 2004.

227. "Scary Strains," *Newsweek*, 1 November 2004.

228. Associated Press, 1 November 2004.

229. Conference press releases: Sabin Vaccine Institute, 28 October; UK government, Health and Community, 23 November; and WHO, Regional Office for Southeast Asia, 25 November 2004.

230. Keith Bradsher and Lawrence Altman, "Tens of Millions," *New York Times*, 29 November 2004.

231. Martin Enserink, "WHO Adds More '1918' to Pandemic Predictions," *Science* 306 (17 December 2004): p. 2025; and Neil Mackay, "Is This the Scourge of 2005?" *Sunday Herald*, 26 December 2004.

232. Richard Webby and Robert Webster, "Are We Ready for Pandemic Influenza?" in Knobler, *Learning from SARS*, p. 217.

233. Quoted in Erika Check, "Thompson Cedes Crown," *Nature* 432 (9 December 2004), p. 660.

234. Robert Pear, "U.S. Health Chief, Stepping Down, Issues Warning," *New York Times*, 4 December 2004.

235. $105 million for abstinence and $100 million for influenza; see *New York Times*, 23 November 2004.

236. Richard Horton, *Heath Wars* (New York: New York Review of Books, 2003), p. 79.

237. GAO.

238. Report quoted in Llewellyn Lefters, Linda Brink, and Ernest Takafuji, "Are We Prepared for a Viral Epidemic Emergency?" in Morse, *Emerging Viruses*, p. 272.

239. Report quoted in Horton, *Heath Wars*, p. 79; and M. Cohen, "Changing Patterns of Infectious Disease," *Nature* 406 (2000): pp. 762–67.

240. Greg Behrman, *The Invisible People* (New York: Free Press, 2004).

241. Government Accounting Office (GAO), *Influenza Pandemic: Plan Needed for Federal and State Response* (Washington, DC: The Office, 2000), pp. 5, 8–11, 17, and 27–28.

242. Institute of Health, *Calling the Shots: Immunization Finance Policies and Practices* (Washington, DC: National Academy Press, 2000), pp. 3–4, 88, and 144.

243. Medical Center, University of Rochester, press release, 12 December 2003.

244. Robert Hockberger, "Even Without a Flu Epidemic, ERs Are in Crisis," *Los Angeles Times*, 27 December 2003.

245. Raymond Strikas, Gregory Wallace, and Martin Myers, "Influenza Pandemic Preparedness Action Plan for the United States: 2002 Update," *CUD* 35 Vaccines (1 September 2002), p. 591.

246. Institute of Medicine, Committee on Assuring the Health of the Public in the 21st Century, *The Future of the Public's Health in the 21st Century* (Washington, DC: National Academy Press, 2003), pp. 97–99.

247. Debora MacKenzie, "Anthrax Attack Bug 'Identical' to Army Strain," *New Scientist*, 9 May 2002.

248. Robert Webster and Elizabeth Walker, "Influenza," *American Scientist* (March–April 2003).

249. Graeme Laver and Robert Webster, "Introduction," *Phil. Trans. R. Soc. Lond.*, 356 B (2001): p. 1814. This message is repeated in Graeme Laver and Elspeth Garman, "The Origin and Control of Pandemic Influenza," *Science* 293 (7 September 2001); Robert Webster and Elizabeth Walker, "Influenza, *American Scientist* (March-April 2003); and Richard Webby and Robert Webster, "Are We Ready for Pandemic Influenza?" *Science* 302 (28 November 2003).

250. Edward Richards, "Bioterrorism and the Use of Fear in Public Health," at http://plague.law.umkc.edu.

Notes

251. U.S. Dept. of Health and Human Services, "Opening Statement by Tommy Thompson, Secretary . . . on Project Bioshield," House Select Commission on Homeland Security, 27 March 2003.

252. Merrill Goozner, "Bioterror Brain Drain," *American Prospect*, 1 October 2003.

253. Scott Shane, "Exposure at Germ Lab Reignites a Public Health Debate," *New York Times*, 24 January 2005.

254. Quoted in Patrick Martin, "US Health Care Workers Spurn Bush Smallpox Vaccination Plan," World Socialist Website (1 March 2003), www.wsws.org.

255. Marcia Angell, *The Truth About the Drug Companies* (New York: Random House, 2004), p. 11.

256. "Drug Makers Find Vaccines Can Be Good for Business," *New York Times*, 29 October 2004.

257. Martin Leeb, "A Shot in the Arm," *Nature* 431 (21 October 2004): p. 893.

258. Greg Critser, "Pharmaceutical Group Chiefs March to Individual Beats," *Los Angeles Times*, 20 December 2000.

259. Donald Barlett and James Steele, "The Health of Nations," *New York Times*, 24 October 2004, Op-Ed.

260. Walsh, "Sickness Spreads," *Time* (Asia), 11 October 2004.

261. Michael Rosenwald, "Flu Crisis Sparks Fresh Look at Vaccine Production," *Washington Post*, 27 November 2004.

262. Halla Thorsteinsdottir, "Cuba—Innovation through Synergy," *Nature Biotechnology* 22 (December 2004): p. DC19.

263. Sabin Russell, *San Francisco Chronicle*, 17 October 2004.

264. Mark Smolinski, Margaret Hamburg, and Joshua Lederberg (eds.), *Microbial Threats to Health: Emergence, Detection and Response*, Institute of Medicine (Washington, DC: National Academies Press, 2003), p. 136.

265. Trust for America's Health, *Ready or Not? Protecting the Public's Health in the Age of Bioterrorism* (Washington, DC: 2004), p. 32.

266. GAO, *Flu Vaccine: Supply Problems Heighten Need to Ensure Access for High-Risk People* (Washington, DC: May 2001); p. 7; and Dr. W. Paul Glezen of Baylor, quoted in *New York Times*, 17 October 2004.

Notes

267. Geoffrey Porges, quoted in Jonathan Peterson and Denise Gellene, "Flu Vaccine Problems Run Deep," *Los Angeles Times*, 18 November 2004.

268. Ibid.

269. Zachary Coile, "Chiron Found Bad Flu Vaccine in July," *San Francisco Chronicle*, 18 November 2004; and David Brown, "U.S. Knew Last Year of Flu Vaccine's Plant's Woes," *Washington Post*, 18 November 2004.

270. Keith Bradsher and Lawrence Altman, "Experts Confront Major Obstacles in Containing Virulent Bird Flu," *New York Times*, 30 September 2004.

271. DHHS, *Draft: Pandemic Influenza Preparedness and Response Plan*, August 2004, p. 23.

272. Editorial, *New York Times*, 12 October 2004.

273. Bradsher and Altman, "Experts."

274. Dr. William Winkenwerder, covering letter to *Department of Defense Pandemic Influenza Preparation and Response Planning Guidance*, office of The Assistant Secretary of Defense, 21 September 2004.

275. Martin Enserink, "Looking the Pandemic in the Eye," *Science* 306 (15 October 2004): p. 394.

276. ACP/ASIM press release, 15 August 2002; and "IDSA Makes Recommendations to Strengthen Draft Plan," *Medical News Today*, 29 October 2004.

277. Quoted in CIDRAP News, 15 November 2004.

278. My emphasis, DHHS, *Draft*, p. 35.

279. Interviewed by Reynolds, "The Flu Hunters," p. 10.

280. John Minz and Joby Warrick, "U.S. Unprepared Despite Progress, Experts Say," *Washington Post*, 8 November 2004.

281. Trust for America's Health, *Ready or Not?*, pp. 3 and 33–34; and *Facing the Flu*, February 2004, pp. 1–2 and 6.

282. Editorial, "Struggling with the Flu," *Nature* 431 (28 October 2004): p. 1023.

283. Kerry-Edwards campaign, "George Bush Passing the Blame on the Flu Vaccine," press release, 19 October 2004.

284. Ralph Nader, "Bush Administration Ignores the Potential Threat of Bird Flu," CommonDreams.org, 4 Feburary 2004; and Nader for President press release, 26 August 2004.

285. Horton, *Heath Wars*, p. 326.

286. Paul Ewald, *Plague Time: The New Germ Theory of Disease* (New York: The Free Press, 2002), pp. 21–25.

287. Paul Ewald, *Evolution of Infectious Disease* (Oxford: Oxford Univ. Press, 1994), pp. 110–13.

288. A. McMichael, "Environmental and Social Influences on Emerging Infectious Diseases: Past, Present and Future," *Phil. Trans. R. Soc. Lond.* 359 B (2004): p. 1052.

289. Ewald, *Evolution*, p. 117.

290. Laurie Garrett, *Betrayal of Trust: The Collapse of Global Public Health* (New York: Hyperion, 2000), pp. 3 and 9.

291. Horton, *Heath Wars*, pp. 325, 328–331, and 343.

292. Editorial, "Political Neglect in India's Health," *Lancet* 363 (15 May 2004): p. 1565.

293. Alex de Waal, "Sex in Summertown," *TLS*, 6 August 2004, p. 6.

294. Vasant Narasimhan et al., "Responding to the Global Human Resources Crisis," *Lancet* 363 (1 May 2004), p. 1469; and *Science* 304 (25 June 2004), p. 1910.

295. Debora MacKenzie, "Lack of Vaccine Raises Fears of Flu Pandemic," NewScientist.com, 23 September 2004; and *Guardian* (London), 23 September 2004.

296. Richard Webby and Robert Webster, "Are We Ready for Pandemic Influenzas?" in Knobler, *Learning from SARS,* p. 214.

297. Kaiser, "Facing Down the Flu," p. 394.

298. Enserink, "Looking," p. 393.

299. Kaiser, "Facing Down the Flu," p. 395.

300. Ibid., p. 397.

301. S. Ragnar Norrby, "Alert to a European Epidemic," *Nature* 431 (30 September 2004): pp. 507–8.

302. Kaiser, "Facing Down the Flu," p. 394.

303. Rene Snacken et al., "The Next Influenza Pandemic: Lessons from Hong Kong, 1997," *Emerging Infectious Diseases* 5, no. 2 (March–April 1999): p. 201.

304. Kaiser, "Facing Down the Flu," p. 394.

305. Bradsher and Altman, "A War and a Mystery."

306. Leeb, "A Shot in the Arm" and Carl Nathan, "Antibiotics at the Crossroads," *Nature* 431 (21 October 2004): pp. 892–93 and 899.

307. Ghanshyam Shah, *Public Health and Urban Development: The Plague in Surat* (New Delhi 1997), pp. 109–10.

308. Garrett, *Betrayal*, p. 27.

309. Ibid., pp. 31–33.

310. Shah, *Urban Development*, pp. 224–26.

311. Kaiser, "Facing Down the Flu," p. 397.

312. "Fact Sheet: HIV/AIDS and the Flu," CDC, 8 November 2004.

313. "Future Flu Epidemic Warning," CBSNEWS.com, 15 December 2004.

314. Keith Bradsher, "Vietnam Seeks Global Aid to Fight Bird Flu," 3 February 2005; and "A Medical Mystery Man Bounces Back from Avian Flu," *New York Times*, 5 February 2005.

315. Quoted in "Vietnam Moves to Curb Bird Flu," *Los Angeles Times*, 3 February 2005.

316. Hans Troedsson and Anton Rychener, "When Influenza Takes Flight," *New York Times*, 5 February 2005, Op-Ed.

317. Pete Aldhous, "Vietnam's War on Flu," *Nature* 433 (13 January 2005): p. 104.

318. "Dangerous State of Denial," *Nature* 433 (12 January 2005).

319. WHO, "Report by the Secretariat: Influenza Pandemic Preparedness and Response," press release, 20 January 2005.

320. CIDRAP News Network, 28 January 2005; and "Secrets and Epidemics," *Los Angeles Times*, 28 January 2005, editorial.

321. Darren Schuettler, "West Urged to Help Fight Avian Flu," *Globe and Mail* (26 February 2005); Menno de Jong, et al., "Fatal Avian Influenza A (H5N1) in a Child Presenting with Diarrhea Followed by a Coma," *New England Journal of Medicine* 352, no. 7 (17 February 2005): p. 686; Barry, *The Great Influenza*, p. 392; and David Syranoski, "Tests in Tokyo Reveal Flaws in Vietnam's Bird Flu Surveillance," *Nature* 433 (24 February 2005): p. 787.

322. Jehangir Pocha, "The Coming Bird Flu Pandemic," *In These Times*, 1 March 2005; and Dennis Normile, "First Human Case in Cambodia Highlights Surveillance Shortcomings," *Science* 307 (18 February 2005).

323. "Avian Influenza: Perfect Storm Now Gathering?" *Lancet* 365 (5 March 2005): p. 820.

324. Martin Enserink and Dennis Normile, "True Numbers Remain Elusive in Bird Flu Outbreak," *Science* 307 (25 March 2005): p. 1865.

325. Rob Stein, "Internal Dissension Grows as CDC Faces Big Threats to Public Health," *Washington Post*, 6 March 2005.

326. Scott Shane, "U.S. Germ-Research Policy is Protested by 758 Scientists," *New York Times*, 1 March 2005.

327. Mike Leavitt, "Preparing Against Pandemic Influenza," (speech text), 7 April 2005 (available at www.medicalnewstoday.com).

328. Shane, "U.S. Germ-Research Policy"; Leavitt, "Preparing Against Pandemic Influenza"; and Gerberding, CIDRAP News, 21 February 2005.

329. *Independent*, 27 Feburary 2005; and Reuters, 2 March 2005.

330. Robert Roos, "Vendor Thought H2N2 Virus was Safe, Officials Say," CIDRAP News, 13 April 2005; "Deadly 1957 Strain of Flu is Found in Lab-Test Kits," Associated Press, 13 April 2005; and Lawrence Altman and Marc Santor, "Risk from Deadly Flu Strain Is Called Low," *New York Times*, 14 April 2005.

331. Roos, "Vendor Thought H2N2 Virus was Safe."

332. OIE press release, 8 April 2005; Alisa Tang, "Bird Flu Strains Could Combine," Associated Press, 6 April 2002; and Dennis Normile, "North Korea Collaborates to Fight Bird Flu," *Science* 308 (8 April 2005).

333. Declan Butler, "Vaccination Will Work Better than Culling, Say Bird Flu Experts," *Nature* 434 (14 April 2005): p. 810.

334. Jeffery Taubenberger et al., "Characterization of the 1918 Influenza Virus Polymerase Genes," *Nature* 437 (6 October 2005): pp. 889–93. On the extraordinary properties of the 1918 virus's HA, see the earlier research by Darwyn Kobasa et al., "Enhanced Virulence of Influenza A Viruses with the Haemagglutinin of the 1918 Pandemic Virus," *Nature* 432 (7 October 2004): pp. 703–7.

335. Betsy McKay, "Avian Virus Caused the 1918 Pandemic," *Wall Street Journal*, 5 October 2005.

336. Andreas von Bubnoff, "The 1918 Flu Virus Is Resurrected," *Nature* 437 (6 October 2005): p. 794.

337. Andreas von Bufnoff, "Deadly Virus Can Be Sent through the Mail," *Nature* 438 (10 November 2005): p. 134.

338. Terrence Tumpey et al., "Characterization of the Reconstructed 1918 Spanish Influenza Pandemic Virus," *Science* 310 (7 October 2005): pp. 77–80. See also Robert Belshe, "The Origins of Pandemic Influenza— Lessons from the 1918 Virus," *New England Journal of Medicine* 353, no. 23 (24 November 2005).

339. Anthony Fauci, "Emerging and Re-emergency Infectious Diseases: Influenza as a Prototype of the Host-Pathogen Balancing Act," *Cell* 124 (24 February 2006): p. 668.

340. Taubenberger et al., p. 892.

341. See contrasting views in Declan Butler, "Yes, but Will It Jump?," *Nature* 439 (12 January 2006): pp. 124–25.

342. "As shown in a virus-binding assay, A/Hong Kong/213/03 infected both alveolar cells and epithelial cells . . ." It is remarkable that none of the press accounts of the Kawaoka research mention this all-important exception. (Kyoko Shinya et al., "Influenza Virus Receptors in the Human Airways," *Nature* 440 (23 March 2006): pp. 435–36.)

343. H. Chen et al., "Establishment of Multiple Sublineages of H5N1 Influenza Virus in Asia: Implications for Pandemic Control," *PNAS* 103, no. 8 (21 February 2006): p. 2849.

344. Ilaria Capua quoted in Martin Enserink, "Veterinary Scientists Shore Up Defenses Against Bird Flu," *Science* 308 (15 April 2005): p. 341.

345. Daphne du Maurier, *The Birds and Other Stories* (London: Virago, 2004, p. 24.

346. A New Zealand ornithologist quoted in David Normile, "Potentially More Lethal Variant Hits Migratory Birds in China," *Science* 309 (8 July 2005): p. 231.

347. Quoted in David Adam, "Avian Flu Found in Migrating Geese," *Guardian,* 7 July 2005.

348. H. Chen et al., "H5N1 Virus Outbreak in Migratory Wildfowl," *Nature* 436 (14 July 2005): p. 191.

349. Dennis Normile, "Chinese Ministry Questions Bird Flu Findings," *Science* 309 (15 July 2005): p. 364.

350. "Chinese Hesitancy on Avian Flu," *Nature* 439 (26 February 2006):

p. 369. See also Keith Bradsher, "Bird Flu," in *New York Times*, 2 February 2006; and Nicholas Zamiska, "How Academic Flap Hurt World Effort on Chinese Bird Flu," *Wall Street Journal*, 24 February 2006.

351. Guan Yi interviewed by Declan Butler in *Nature* 440 (6 April 2006): p. 727.

352. E-mail exchanges (researcher anonymous).

353. David Holley, "Bird Flu Besieges Southern Russia," *Los Angeles Times*, 2 March 2006.

354. "The majority of Nigeria's chickens live in and around people's homes, so risks of human exposure and disease are high." Martin Enserink, "H5N1 Moves into Africa, European Union, Deepening Global Crisis," *Science* 311 (17 February 2006): p. 932.

355. E-mail conversations with Robert Wallace, University of California at Irvine.

356. Marius Gilbert et al., "Free-grazing Ducks and Highly Pathogenic Avian Influenza, Thailand," *Emerging Infectious Diseases* 12, no. 2 (February 2006): p. 227.

357. Infected poultry in southern China, however, remain the principal biological reservoir of H5N1. See H. Chen et al., "Establishment of Multiple Sublineages of H5N1 Influenza Virus in Asia: Implications for Pandemic Control," *PNAS* 103, no. 8 (21 February 2006): pp. 2845–50.

358. Dennis Normile, "Evidence Points to Migratory Birds in H5N1 Spread," *Science* 311 (3 March 2006): p. 1225.

359. A. Dennis Lemly, Richard Kingsford, and Julian Thompson, "Irrigated Agriculture and Wildlife Conservation: Conflict on a Global Scale," *Environmental Management* 25, no. 5 (2000): p. 498. Alternatively, some experts argue that smuggled poultry may have been the source of the outbreak in northern Nigeria. (Elizabeth Rosenthal, "Bird Flu Virus May Be Spread By Smuggling," *New York Times*, 15 April 2006.)

360. United Nations Environment Programme (Nairobi), "Restoration of Wetlands Key to Reducing Future Threats of Avian Flu," press release, 11 April 2006.

361. E-mail note from Jeremijenko; also Declan Butler, "Can Cats Spread Avian Flu?" *Nature* 440 (9 March 2006): p. 135.

362. "Experts Urge Including Cats in Avian Flu Precautions," *CIDRAP*

News (5 April 2006); and Carter Dougherty, "Bird Flu Fears and New Rules Rattle German Pet Lovers," *New York Times*, 5 March 2006.

363. Butler, ibid.; and Albert Osterhuas et al., "Feline Friend or Potential Foe?," *Nature* 440 (6 April 2006): pp. 741–42.

364. Ricardo Alonso-Zaldivar, "Bird Flu Strain Expected to Land in U.S. This Year," *Los Angeles Times,* 14 March 2006.

365. See "H5N1 Vaccine Trial Shows Limited Benefit," *CIDRAP News* (30 March 2006); and Grefory Poland, "Vaccines aginst Avian Influenza—A Race against Time," *New England Journal of Medicine* 354, no. 13 (March 30, 2006): pp. 1411–13.

366. The same nineteen experts gave a median estimate of 15 percent for avian flu to acquire a pandemic mutation within the same period. The Carnegie Mellon study by Wandi De Bruin and Baruch Fischhoff cited in "U.S. Unlikely to Have Enough Vaccines to Stop Avian Flu Pandemic," *RxPG News* (22 March 2006).

Index

acute respiratory infection, 24
Afkhami, Amir, 29–30
Africa: influenza in, 23–24;
  pandemic fears for, 162–63; public
  health in, 156–57, 163
Agriculture Department, 91
AIDS, 55, 56, 58, 129, 130, 163
amantadine, 112
American College of Physicians,
  146
American Expeditionary Force, 30
American Medical Association, 25
American Samoa, 33
American Society of Internal
  Medicine, 146
American Spectator (journal), 100
Andrewes, Christopher, 34
Andromeda Strain, The (Crichton), 5
Angell, Marcia, 137
anthrax, 133, 135
antibiotics, 138, 160, 162
antigenic drift, 11, 16, 38
antigenic shift, 11, 17

antiviral medications, stockpiling of,
  131, 134–35, 144, 159–60
Armed Forces Institute of Pathology,
  Maryland, 118
Asian flu (1957), 16, 35–36
Australia, 33
Aventis-Pasteur, 124, 140, 141, 147,
  158
avian flu: deadliness of, 7, 126; first
  human appearance of, 4; genetic
  mutation in, 7–8, 11–12, 15, 63–67;
  as global plague, 4; globalization
  and, 8; in Guangdong, China,
  58–67; in Hong Kong, 45–54;
  human-to-human transmission of,
  120; person-to-person transmission
  of, 7–8; poultry industry and, 108;
  propagation of, 9–10; research on,
  38, 116–18; in Thailand, 101–14;
  treatment of, 7, 19; 2003
  reappearance of, 5, 101–14. *See also*
  Highly Pathogenic Avian Influenza
  (HPAI)

Index

Index

Index

Index

Administration (FDA), 42, 127–28, 140, 142–44; Health and Human Services Department (HHS), 128–33, 137, 140–41, 144, 146; 1918 flu pandemic in, 26, 32; preparedness for influenza pandemic in, 128–38, 143–50; public health system inadequacy in, 128–33, 147–48; vaccines for influenza in, 129–31, 134–50

urban poverty, 8, 28–29, 55–56, 152–54

Urbani, Carlo, 71

vaccines: Cuba and, 139–40; flu caused by, 102; Franics/Salk, 34; free enterprise and control of, 35–38, 41–42, 129–30, 144; global strategy for, 123–24; global supply of, 157–60; immunization programs, 42, 44, 156; new technologies for, 139, 158; pharmaceutical industry reluctance to develop, 8, 41–42, 44, 124, 129, 137, 139–41; problems in manufacturing, 139–40, 142–43; public policy on, 37–38, 41–44, 129–31, 134–36, 144–49, 159–60; rationing of, 135, 143, 145–46; SARS, 76; smallpox, 135; stockpiling of, 19, 123–24, 135, 145; UNICEF spending on, 156; unprofitability of, 138; updating, 34; U.S. and, 129–31, 134–50

Van Dongen, John, 95

veterinary medicine, 89

Viagra, 138

Vietnam, 75–76, 103–4, 108, 111–14, 119, 157, 160

Vietnam News (newspaper), 108

Vioxx, 128

viral diseases: animal-human transmission of, 58; globalization as context for, 55–67

Viraphol, Sarasin, 105

Washington Post (newspaper), 147–48

Waxman, Henry, 42, 142

Webby, Richard, 21, 63, 127

Webster, Robert, 15, 21, 48–49, 55, 77, 95, 112, 116, 127, 134–35, 141, 145

Weiss, Robin, 69

West Africa, 57–58

wet markets, 45, 59, 75

Wickramasinghe, Chandra, 15n

wildlife trade, viral diseases spread through, 60, 75–76

Wolfe, Nathan, 58

World Health Organization (WHO), 7, 23; criticisms of, 156; and Dutch avian flu (2003), 88; global influence of, 156; and Hong Kong avian flu (1997), 51, 60–61, 67; influenza fears of, 4, 123–26, 150, 151, 162–63; and pharmaceutical industry, 156; and pneumonic plague in India, 162; and SARS,

World Health Organization (WHO)
(continued)
69–76, 78; on transmissibility of
avian flu, 118; and 2004
reappearance of avian flu, 119–21;
and 2003 reappearance of avian
flu, 104, 110–14; on vaccine
needs, 158–60; vaccine stockpile
for, 19, 123–24; world influenza
network established by, 24, 34–35
World War I, 31–32, 151–52

World War II, 33–34
Wyeth, 41
Wyeth-Ayerst, 140

Yanzhong Huang, 59, 73–75
Young India (newspaper), 28
Yukol Limlamthong, 120

Zambia, 157
zanamivir (Relenza), 19, 134n
Zhang Wenkang, 73, 74